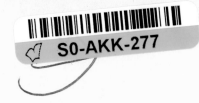

The complete book of acupuncture

The complete book
of acupuncture

Dr. Stephen Thomas Chang

Preface by Dolph B. Ornstein M.D.

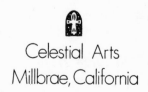

Celestial Arts
Millbrae, California

Illustrations by Mary Elizabeth Bruno

CELESTIAL ARTS
231 Adrian Road
Millbrae, California 94030

First Printing, September 1976
Made in the United States of America

Library of Congress Cataloging in Publication Data

Chang, Stephen Thomas, 1935–
    The complete book of acupuncture.

    Includes index.
    1. Acupuncture. I. Title. [DNLM; 1. Acupuncture.
WB369 C39c]
RM184.C4814   615'.892   75-28762
ISBN 0-89087-124-8

1 2 3 4 5 6 7 – 81 80 79 78 77 76

PREFACE

A new day is dawning, an awareness to the truth is growing, the times indeed are changing. But how does this affect the medical profession and the delivery of an effective health care system?

One measure of the wisdom and perhaps the major criteria of a "successful" society is the health and happiness of its peoples—for all suffer or benefit from one's beliefs which are intrinsically part of our culture.

Our view of ourselves and of our society is rapidly changing. The nature of reality and the concept of what is real is undergoing a dramatic change—we are probing into our subconscious collective selves; we are discovering individually and collectively fascinating aspects and mechanisms which govern our existence. We are beginning to understand the natural laws which rule the universe and ourselves of which we are intimately a part.

Many perceive these changes and are fearful of them because they appear to be responsible for much of the chaos and disorder which is regularly broadcast on the daily news. However, revolution and evolution cannot be separated, for revolutionary ideas and concepts, when understood and internalized by man, create something new, something greater, something more profound.

It has been said that the only constant is change; with change comes "death" followed by rebirth. "Death" is really but an acceptance that the old system of thought (and hence our beliefs) does not truly explain the phenomenon of life. We try desperately to maintain our beliefs because they afford us a structure, a form, a reason for being—and enormous security in a world which appears to be increasingly dangerous and bewildering. We are kept in bondage, however, because in each and every one of us there is a titanic struggle to emerge free, to express ourselves for what we are, regardless of what we are. We are all striving consciously or subconsciously for our own personal truths, for the truth shall set us free; but the truth cannot be intellectualized nor can it be debated, it can only be experienced and felt and because it is the truth it can be observed and perceived.

It is remarkable today to see how the psychiatrists and the physicists are moving, however hesitantly, toward similar unifying concepts to explain the phenomenon which we call life; concepts which in the past were belittled as occultism, mysticism or other such doctrines which were bereft of intellectual debate. Yet one has only to look and study to note a glorious connecting thread in all the great works of art and philosophies of man through the ages both Eastern and Western. The great theoretical physicists see the cosmos mathematically; the great artists express themselves in the forms of sound, movement, color and music, all of which can be understood mathematically.

Hence, a discussion of medicine must include philosophy, for to deny this is to deny the fact that the body exacts an influence over the mind and the mind exacts an influence over the body. It has been said that the body is but a reflection and manifestation of the mind. This can be easily understood if one examines the gait and appearance of a joyous, happy person as compared with one who is depressed and unhappy. On the other hand, a body which is sick or injured or in pain exerts its influence over the mind in the form of unpleasant emotions. What is the determinant between these two poles, the happy or positive and the unhappy or negative? The determinant of course is the level of energy, for it is energy which sustains everything.

Since it is energy which sustains and manifests itself in an infinite variety of forms it is also the intensity of energy or the relative lack of it which sustains our health or detracts from it.

The unifying concept in my mind is that the Universe, or cosmos, is in a state of dynamic equilibrium, constantly changing, undergoing "death" only to resurrect itself into life and creativity once again, thus continuing the vortex in a never ending cycle of life, "death" and rebirth; and what is true for the cosmos is true for ourselves. The *Taoist* concept upon which acupuncture is based, states "as is above, so is below." Also inherent in Taoist thought is the concept of microcosm and macrocosm, with man being the microcosm within an awesome macrocosm which sustains us. Each cell within our bodies is a miniature universe which sustains itself for the good of the whole and it is the whole which provides energy for the functioning of the cells.

What does this have to do with man and his medicine today? Well, quite simply, *everything* because we as Western doctors have, through a superficial system of thought and belief, alienated ourselves. We do not deal with universal principles because we cannot perceive them nor can we detect them, and because we do not acknowledge them we deny their existence. To deny the flow and ebb of life, to deny the sense of spirit, the transmutability of all things, is to be blind and this blindness manifests itself in a form of medicine which tyrannizes us all. It is because we do not deal on a day-to-day level with the profound reality of life that we daily invite and court personal havoc and disarray. Medical science is steeped in the philosophy of scientific materialism; we have lost the awareness of the interconnectedness of all things and fail to recognize important relationships within the body. Only now are medical researchers beginning to acknowledge the existence of an "aura"—a field of electromagnetism which exudes from the physical body. But this same aura has been depicted through the ages in innumerable works of *art*.

It is the Taoist concept that *dis-ease* is the result of an energy imbalance and the spectrum extends from total madness (Dante's *Inferno*) to an exuberance and exaltation which words cannot describe (Dante's *Paradise*). Thus, feeling good means different things to different people. We quite readily accept those vague feelings of ill-will as part of our birthright. We have deluded ourselves into thinking that this is the way life is. But we must understand, if we are to change and to move to greater health, that we do indeed "reap what we sow" and that health is a reflection of balance, and balance is the sum total of how we live.

As noted before, Western medicine is based on a philosophical concept of scientific rational materialism; it directs its energies toward overt disease entities and a classification system which creates enormous separations. If one were to step back and make a truly scientific non-emotional evaluation of where we are *now* as regards the collective health of this nation and its practice of medicine, one would inevitably be led to the sad conclusion that in many instances we are creating more harm than good.

One of the cardinal rules of medicine, as I was taught, is: physician, *do no harm.* Respect the body. Understand that the body has fabulous healing potential of its own and this constant insulting of the body with harsh chemicals and often brutal surgical procedures creates emotional and physical disasters. We so often engage in vigorous therapy for disease entities of which we have no substantial understanding. The entire emphasis of Western medicine is negativistic in that it only diagnoses disease states which have become manifest in innumerable entities to which we apply words which often convey nothing as to what is really happening. What does *systemic lupus erythematosis* mean? What is it? It is a description of an entity of which the causes are totally unknown.

It should be understood that the individual has the ability to create within himself innumerable possibilities; hence, one has only to read a pathology text book to see how creative we are in a negativistic way.

I want to emphasize that the basic direction of Chinese medicine is toward *prevention* and should an imbalance occur with a resultant disease, acupuncture is employed to restore the body and mind to an equilibrium which we call health. Another essential point to be made is that acupuncture is based on *scientific principles* and introduces a new concept we in the West are just beginning to recognize as valid. The Chinese, through 6,000 years of trial and error, have come to know that the body possesses a meridian system which basically is electromagnetic currents circulating through the body. These meridians are connected through the skin to various organ systems, the relationships of which are *not* understood in the West.

It is through this meridian system that the organ systems are stimulated in order to effect change. All diseases are the result of energy blocks or imbalances which manifest into innumerable disturbances which have plagued mankind throughout the ages. Cancer, rheumatoid arthritis and diabetes are but a few of the entities which are thoroughly understood and treatable diseases within the construct and concepts of Chinese medicine.

While many of us in the West are not clinically sick (in that we do not have overt disease) we are plagued by feelings of mild depression which are enigmatic for the practicing doctor. A patient comes to the clinic or office complaining of malaise, tiredness, weariness or listlessness; a battery of tests is done to rule out known clinical entities. Most of the time our laboratory results are unfruitful. We label these systems as either psychosomatic or neurotic (note the use of words which convey nothing except to say that we are unable to deal with the problems effectively because we know that these problems are deeply rooted and reflect a person's life style and various emotional problems). We are at a loss to treat such an individual effectively because generally it is the person's life circumstances and tendencies which have created his situation. The general mode of treatment is a quick pep talk and perhaps some antihypertensive medicine or a tranquilizer and the patient is sent on his way to deal as best he can with the tensions and anxieties with which each and everyone of us is confronted daily. If the patient is insistent enough he may be referred to a psychiatrist where an attempt is made to elucidate the causes of the stressful situation. This can often be a long and arduous journey with considerable expense and with no guarantee of success.

Chinese philosophy and medicine approach the problem differently. A basic aspect of Chinese medical philosophy is that the person himself is responsible for his or her own health and it is the role of the physician to be a teacher or guide. However, in times of serious imbalances the physician now elucidates the cause and the treatment depends on what is found; it is tailored to the particular needs of the patient. *In other words, the treatment is not standardized, it is individualized.* This is an essential difference between the Western medical approach and Chinese medicine and reflects the incredible art and sensitivity of Chinese medicine.

The experienced acupuncturist can diagnose the imbalance at the wrist. The doctor tells you where the problem lies and what is needed to resolve the problem. The treatment varies as noted according to the degree of pathology. Often, the treatment is just herbs (i.e. nutritional), and oftentimes it is acupressure and acupuncture or a combination of herbs, acupressure, acupuncture and *good common sense.*

Another facet of Chinese medicine not generally known in the West is an entire system of Internal Exercises to nourish and prevent diseases of organ systems. I view this as a form of Chinese yoga.

To complete the holistic approach to health and happiness, the Chinese long ago addressed themselves to the problems and potentials of human sexuality. It is obvious to all that a healthy, exciting sexual life greatly enhances our appreciation of ourselves and of the world. To express our human love completely to another has always been man's deepest desire. Love is energy and it sustains all things.

For balance and good health to be maintained, we need to learn more about our sexual energies because it is the abuse and often the negation of these energies which create many, if not all, of man's anxieties and tensions. A healthy, more balanced view of our sexuality is an inherent part of the holistic concept exposed by Taoist thought and conceived in Chinese medical doctrine. Thus, what we have in terms of medical practice is a system which deals with the mind and the body as a unit, each influencing and dependent upon the other.

If the concepts and the techniques are grasped, one can plainly see that all diseases, both mental and physical, may be treated. The limitations and frustrations of Western medicine are well known to the public and professionals alike. The major diseases which afflict our society such as cancer, rheumatoid arthritis, atherosclerotic heart disease, diabetes mellitus, cancer, hypertension, migraines, low back pain, hyperthyroidism, hypothyroidism, anxiety, depression, impotence, schizophrenia, insomnia, epilepsy, disseminated sclerosis, chronic pain syndrome, the common cold, menstrual irregularities, emphysema, asthma, myopia, cataracts, ulcerative colitis, irritable bowel syndrome, hemorrhoids, Crohn's disease, appendicitis, hyperactivity in children, hepatitis, nephritis, pneumonitis, cystitis, venereal infestations, duodenal and peptic ulceration, disseminated lupus erythematosus, rheumatism, myalgia, alcoholism, and heroin addictions are all manifestations of varying degrees of energy imbalances. (The list above is not comprehensive.) It is toward the balancing of these imbalances that Chinese medical practice directs its energies.

I find acupuncture and its attendant medical philosophies so exciting because many of the above insights have been noted, recorded and understood through the ages; however, an attendant practical system has not accompanied these grandiose concepts.

Many books have appeared on the market discussing acupuncture. However, as is well known, any great truth or system, if not truly understood, can be misapplied and distorted. Dr. Chang is a direct descendant of a long line of Chinese physicians. His great-grandfather was physician to an Empress of China. This work is a direct translation from Chinese manuscripts to English. Nothing is being lost in adaptation or in translation. Dr. Chang, in the spirit of humility and love, wants to share what he knows with us so that we collectively can try to alleviate the suffering and pain which is so prevalent in our world today.

Acupuncture is a science and deserves the time and patience of any new discipline to be understood and mastered. It is a creative art as well because medicine is indeed a healing art. One cannot learn acupuncture in four or six weeks. It is just this impatience, which is so characteristic of our way of life, which negates a true understanding of this wonderful system and which also negates its full potential. It is and would be a great mistake to shut ourselves off from a healing system which is time proven, non-invasive and eminently in tune with the nature of reality. As was the case in Isiah's day, so it is today, "where there is no vision, the people perish."

We have always had the power to effect change. Hopefully, we will grasp some of these ideas and concepts and move toward a more positive approach to life and medicine—as always, the choice is ours.

DOLPH B. ORNSTEIN, M.D.

CONTENTS

INTRODUCTION

Within the past few years, the science of acupuncture has captured the interest of both professionals and laymen throughout America. This interest initially began as a result of former President Richard Nixon's trip to China and immediately many people began to regard acupuncture as something miraculous—a panacea for all ills. Unfortunately, the phenomenal claims attributed to this science were to its disadvantage, for the over-expectant imaginations of its supporters caused the techniques of this ancient science to be applied without practitioners first acquiring a thorough understanding of its basic theories and practices. I personally knew of some "doctors" who claimed to be treating up to 60 patients per day, and their patients, in some instances, actually had to stand in a long line outside the door of the doctor's small office. In the rush and hurry so characteristic of the Western way of life, these new advocates of acupuncture had not allowed themselves enough time to study and thoroughly assimilate all aspects of acupuncture therapy. It was inevitable then, in the course of time, that the delusions sustained by the fanatical claims of many of the over-enthusiastic supporters of this ancient science would ultimately be shattered.

The scientific and philosophical system upon which acupuncture is built cannot be assimilated overnight; for the effective application of acupuncture, the subtle thought processes must be modified in accordance with scientific principles as expounded in acupuncture philosophy. These scientific principles are the outcome of a cultural-philosophical system that offers a different explanation of man and life than that to which Westerners are accustomed; and when they are applied, they often confuse the Westerner. It is no wonder then that acupuncture has become a highly controversial subject, for Westerners have simply assumed that it can be applied without giving any consideration to the different cultural system upon which it is based.

At present, acupuncture holds the interest of many laymen, but professionals are divided as to its effectiveness. The reasons that were first published as to the ineffectiveness of acupuncture motivated me to come to the defense of this form of therapy that I have practiced for over 20 years.

There are three main objections to the acceptance of acupuncture. They are:

1. Acupuncture does not work.
2. Acupuncture offers only temporary relief and does not cure.
3. Acupuncture is dangerous because it temporarily stops the pain which is a warning signal not to be ignored.

The first objection—acupuncture does not work—is the result of a very superficial acquaintance with the science. Simply the test of time itself, upon which the validation of many a scientific and philosophical system is based, would put the science of acupuncture on a level absolutely unsurpassed by many of the other totally accepted sciences and philosophies; it has existed for over 5,000 years.

It is only in the past few decades that many of the theories of acupuncture, that had been labeled purely philosophical and impossible to validate under scientific conditions, have been verified as a result of technological advancements in laboratory equipment enabling scientists to verify the subtler aspects of this ancient healing system. Thorough study of this ancient science under the guidance of one who is an experienced practitioner will dispel all erroneous ideas connected with its system.

In regard to the second objection—that acupuncture offers only temporary relief and does not actually cure—several factors must be considered first to understand the basis for this objection and, at the same time, to demonstrate the inherent error in those factors.

Unlike Western medical doctors, a practitioner of acupuncture is advised only to treat a maximum of eight patients a day. It is impossible to effect a complete cure of any illness without spending a minimum of one hour with each patient. By haphazardly inserting needles into patients and immediately removing them, one may diminish the intensity of specific pains, but no complete cure is guaranteed. Inserting a needle and immediately removing it is actually a *Dispersal Technique*—energy is lost rather than gained; if one is unaware of this, the ultimate effect will be fatal. The age-old saying "haste makes waste" is especially true in regard to acupuncture treatment. True, temporary relief is all that will result if the quantity of the patients seen, rather than the quality of treatment administered, is the motivating factor in a practitioner.

Before treating any patient a lengthy *Diagnosis* is necessary; a hasty diagnosis is a sure indication that treatment will be unsuccessful. One of the most important steps of *Diagnosis, Reading the Pulse,* requires a minimum of three years experience. My files are filled with innumerable cases of "incurable" diseases that have been cured by acupuncture once the fundamentals of *Diagnosis* are understood and mastered.

In regard to the third objection—that acupuncture relieves pain, and thus the patient neglects to receive treatment for their disease—my many years of experience in conjunction with both Chinese and Japanese doctors has led me to the acceptance of a new theory concerning the relationship between pain and disease.

Several years ago I was given the opportunity of treating a man afflicted with lung cancer. His pain was terribly intense and he had been given the maximum amount of morphine it was possible to give—nothing else was possible, death seemed imminent. After the first treatment of acupuncture, his pain was reduced by about 30 percent. After 14 treatments over a three-week period, the pain was completely stopped. At the same time, X-rays revealed the cancer area had become much smaller than before. The man returned home from the hospital. After another 14 treatments, X-rays showed the midus was much smaller and dry. I concluded that, by diminishing the intensity of a patient's pain through acupuncture, his body's energy is restored and able to combat the focus of disease, rather than being dispelled through his anguish.

In another instance, I treated a woman who could not turn her neck and who had been taking pain pills and physical therapy for three years. During this three-year period she had not slept more than two hours at a time because of the pain. After only one acupuncture treatment she slept seven hours— the most sleep she had gotten in three years. This woman eventually recovered and stopped taking pain pills because her body energy was no longer dissipated in coping with the pain.

I would also like to mention the case of that concerning a 33-year-old man who had been consulting a dermatologist for two years and six months. He had small blister type sores on the glans of his penis that had been diagnosed as the result of a venereal disease. The sores were painful to touch and despite all antibiotics, salves, and injections, they persisted. A series of tests revealed that the initial infection had not been completely destroyed by the antibiotics and it was believed that the remaining bacteria had confined themselves to the cells of the skin tissue to which the capillaries had no access. It was finally concluded that he had a specific strain of venereal disease that was immune to all forms of treatment.

After 14 acupuncture treatments, those symptoms that had persisted for the two and a half years disappeared. I believe that the germs were destroyed by his own body power (or energy) which was augmented through specific acupuncture techniques.

Finally, I treated a man who had chronic bronchitis and initial asthma. He also had severe pain in the back and chest. His pain had plagued him for seven years! After three periods of treatments (36 acupuncture treatments), all of his pain had disappeared and has not reappeared for additional treatment within the past year.

Hundreds of cases demonstrate that once the painful symptoms are relieved, the energy that is no longer being dissipated in coping with those symptoms can restore the body to its original state of health.

One of my purposes in writing this book is to give the reader a general knowledge of the basic principles and techniques of this ancient science. Acupuncture must be considered in its totality, for it is not the kind of science that can be compartmentalized in such a way that a person can become a "specialist" in one branch of the entire field it encompasses. One who aspires to become a practitioner must learn to view the body in its entirety, and the concept of entirety rules out specification.

I sincerely feel that this book, in comparison to all the others now available is the most thorough and complete. Whether one is interested in merely acquainting himself with basic principles and practices, or actually applying those practices on himself to increase his vitality and regain his youth, this book will be of value.

It is hoped that the knowledge contained within this book will enable man to free himself from the limitations of disease and attain a truly perfect state of health that will benefit the generations to come. To this noble task this book is dedicated.

DR. STEPHEN T. CHANG
San Francisco, California

PART I

The Basic Knowledge of Acupuncture

FOREWORD

Part I of this book deals with the basic philosophy of acupuncture included in which are the energy theory, the law of the five elements, the meridians, the organs and bowels, biorhythm, diagnostic procedures, and various modes of therapy such as needling, meridian massage, and application of moxa. In order to acquire an understanding of any of these vital subjects it will be necessary to go beyond merely reading about them and actually experience them, for scholarship—as laudable as it may be—is of no great value if that knowledge cannot be practically applied to one's own personal growth and to the growth of others. To both read and experience are therefore necessary if you wish to develop that sense of discriminative creativity so absolutely necessary to the beneficent application of acupuncture techniques.

A thorough understanding of subjects such as the meridian system and the concept of the flow of energy can be acquired while simultaneously developing an expertise at acupressure and massage by massaging the entire length of each meridian in the direction of the flow of energy; in this way a purely intellectual understanding of these subjects is reinforced by actually experiencing them. Eventually as you become more aware of the energy within your own body as a result of these practices, you will be able to realize the validity of the subtle biorhythm cycles as they relate to the circulation of energy

1

throughout your own body. Reading the pulses—a standard diagnostic procedure—can be attempted with a greater chance of success as you become aware of your own body energy and how its balance is reflected at the radial artery of the wrist.

Acupuncture is a subjective science in that it is, in the deepest sense of the word, an art. Like any other art, its effective expression is dependent upon the cultivation of an inner creative genius ever growing from a firm foundation—the basic principles of this ancient science.

Acupuncture is as much a medical science as it is an art; but it is not the type of science that is simply studied and mechanically applied using, as an example, the same prescription for the common cold for every person with a common cold. Acupuncture can justifiably be called a marriage between science and art in that its time-tested, prescribed therapies, while based on firmly established scientific principles, are not rigidly applied; each can and—in many cases—must be modified in the light of your inner creativity and awareness of the distinctively individual needs of each person.

WHAT IS ACUPUNCTURE?

Acupuncture is a therapy used for the prevention of disease or for the maintenance of health. The practice consists of either stimulating or dispersing the flow of energy within the body by the insertion of needles into specific points on the surface of the skin, by applying heat (thermal therapy), by pressing, by massage, or by a combination of these. Acupuncture was developed by the Chinese, and its origins date back almost 6000 years.

NEEDLES

Style and type of needles:

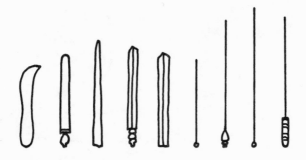

FIGURE 1. *Nine needles.*

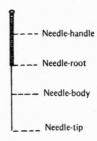

FIGURE 2. *At the present time, No. 32 1-tsun (Chinese inch) needles are generally used.*

APPLICATION OF HEAT—MOXIBUSTION (THE BURNING OF MOXA)

Moxibustion is a thermal therapy in which an herb called *moxa* (*Artemisia vulgaris, Artemisia argyi L'evl et Vant*) is placed upon a chosen point on the skin's surface and ignited; it is left to burn all the way down to the skin, is frequently painful and produces a blister. Some people, however, report that the burning will actually cause a pleasant sensation, in all probability due to the increase of circulation around the point being treated. A very thin slice of ginger placed between the moxa and the skin will diminish the intensity of the pain and also the severity of the blister. Moxa can be purchased in the forms of pyramids (cones), long sticks, and most recently, moxa-rolls.

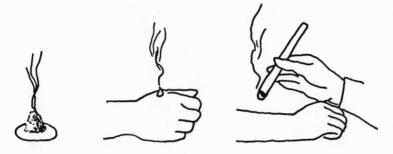

FIGURE 3. *Moxibustion.*

ACUPRESSING (YAH-HSUEH)

The thumbs and palms are used to apply pressure to specific points on the surface of the skin. Before applying acupressure or massage it is advised that the hands be briskly rubbed together until a definite sensation of warmth is felt in the palms. The pulsating warmth resulting from the friction of rubbing the hands together indicates an increase of energy that should be willfully directed into the acupuncture points in the vicinity of affected areas of the body.

The beneficial effects of laying-on-of-hands, a spiritual healing technique utilized by innumerable religions throughout the ages, are readily explainable in that the energy flowing throughout the body is "reversed" in the hands and fingers, and therefore the hands are saturated with magnetic charges that can be directed into affected body areas by a trained will. Recent Kirlian photography techniques have demonstrated the mind's ability to affect the energy that emanates from within the body.

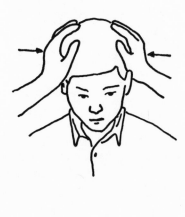

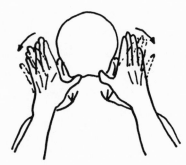

FIGURE 4. *Acupressing.*

MASSAGE (TUI-NAH)

Meridian Digital Pressure is actually the correct name for this form of massage which is very different from occidental massage in that it focuses primarily upon stimulating the flow of basic energy within the body rather than simply relieving muscular tension.

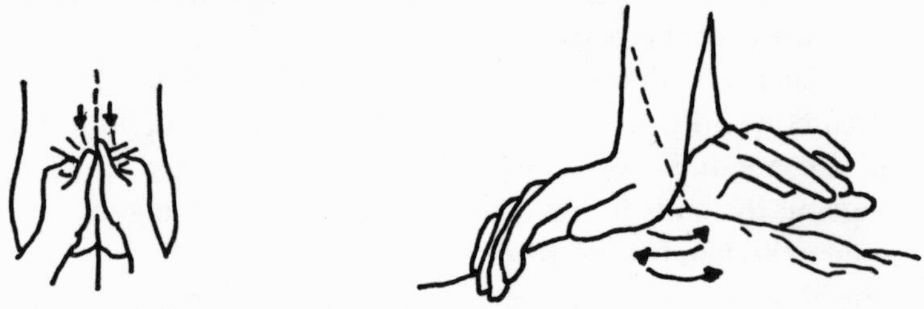

FIGURE 5. *Massage* (Tui-nah).

2

WHY ACUPUNCTURE WORKS

THE INHERENCY THEORY

The human body has a miraculous power to regenerate and repair itself. For instance: scraped skin will grow back in a few days without any conscious effort on the part of an individual; if a morsel of food or some water accidentally goes into the trachea, the person will automatically cough to expel the foreign substance; if a small particle of dirt or dust gets in the eye, tears immediately begin to wash the particle away. These are only a few of the many ways in which the body works to restore the equilibrium once it has been disturbed. Inherent within the life force is the tendency to sustain itself and maintain a perfect balance within the body under all circumstances.

Chinese medicine encourages people to become aware of the miraculous powers inherent within their bodies and to takeadvantage of these powers before they rely on outside aid. Hippocrates, the father of medicine, said that nature is medicine and that medicine is the servant of nature. The people who coined the proverb, "Nature cures the illness, but the doctor gets the fee," were thinking along the same lines.

Acupuncture is a therapy that has been used by the Chinese people to stimulate or awaken the natural power within the body. In the course of time people have lost confidence in, and even the awareness of, their self-healing powers. As their awareness of their own healing potentials has become dimmed, they have become dependent upon chemical drugs and injections.

THE ENERGY THEORY

According to the Chinese hypothesis, the body is endowed with a definite energy quotient at birth. While this energy is being dissipated through the *vicissitudes* of daily living, it is simultaneously being replenished by energy obtained from food and air (included within air is the all-pervading electro-magnetic energy). Energy imbalance—either an excess or an insufficiency—is the root of all illness; total absence of energy is death.

Energy is believed to circulate throughout the body in well defined cycles; moving in a prescribed sequence from organ to bowel via the meridians, it flows partly at the periphery and partly in the interior of the body. Energy within the body is considered to be a dynamic force in constant flux; this is a leading principle in Chinese medicine, an important hypothesis within the framework of which the empirical theory of acupuncture was developed. The energy theory as being the basis for the effective application of acupuncture is explained in greater detail in Chapter 4.

THE BLOOD THEORY

After conducting an extensive series of experiments in which rats and rabbits were used as subjects, the following phenomenon were revealed:

Vasodilation. After sedating a rabbit, an incision was made in the abdomen and a portion of the large intestine was firmly fixed under a microscope. Needles were inserted into specific points on the dorsal side of the neck and into the chest. Vasodilation immediately occurred and continued for as long as the needles remained intact. This led to the conclusion that acupuncture could promote an increased blood circulation among the organs, especially those of the digestive system.

Vasoconstriction. A series of experiments were conducted in which rats were used. Needles were inserted into specific points on the back and especially along the spinal column. Vasoconstriction within the brain immediately occurred and continued as long as the needles remained intact. This led to the conclusion that acupuncture could help relieve apoplexy and could also be applied to regulate the blood pressure.

Blood Increase. Regardless of the prevailing state of health, after inserting needles into specific points on the body, blood tests revealed that the white corpuscles and neutrophil juvenile had markedly increased. Coagulase, fibrin, hemolysin and serum also increased. The increase in the percentage of white corpuscles led to the conclusion that acupuncture could enable the body to effectively combat strains of infectious disease that had developed an immunity to antibiotics such as penicillin.

THE NERVE THEORY

Thousands of years ago Chinese physicians began to meticulously observe the nervous system within the body. Eventually they discovered that the nerves provided a pathway for nerve impulses generated in response to both internal and external environmental changes. They also discovered that the meridians were pathways that provided for the circulation of energy throughout the body. Later it was found that both systems were interrelated. Figure 6 illustrates the acupuncture points on the posterior side of the body that exist along the spinal column. A needle inserted into these points will affect the corresponding spinal nerve that stems from the spinal column and travels to a visceral organ.

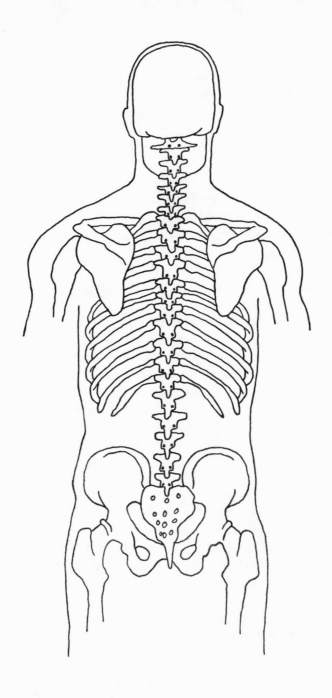

Figure 6. *Acupuncture points affecting the spinal nerves.*

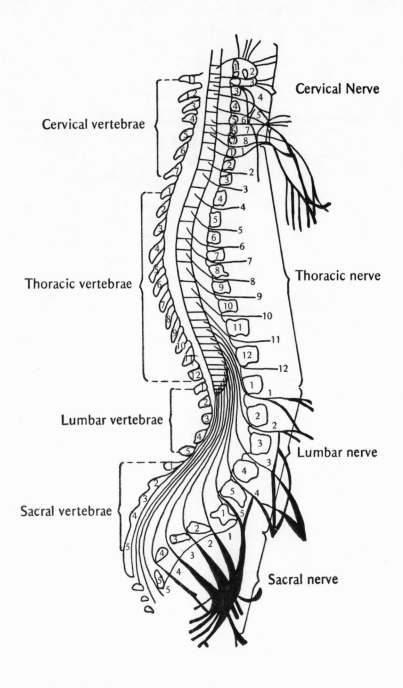

FIGURE 7. *Diagram of the spinal nerves.*

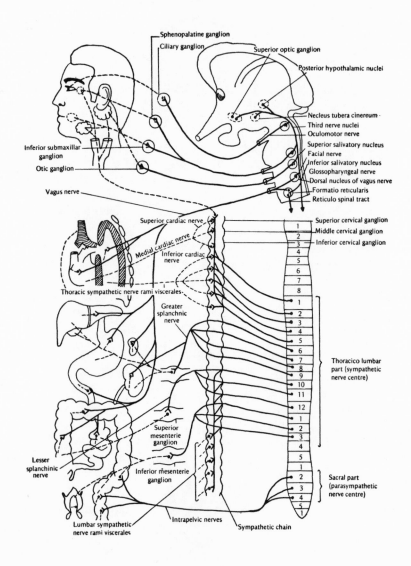

FIGURE 8. *A diagram of the efferent nerves of the internal organs.*
12

In coping with pain, acupuncture has been utilized in the following ways: First, pain can be alleviated by inserting needles into points that will affect an afferent nerve (a nerve that stems from an internal viscera that conveys pain, sensations of hunger, sex, etc.) and block the impulse from reaching the brain. Second, by inserting needles into points that will affect an afferent nerve an impulse can be generated that will preoccupy the nerve center in the brain. The nerve center being preoccupied with the surrogate impulse fails to attend to the original pain that has become secondary and which will eventually subside. The primary purpose of generating a surrogate impulse is to enable the energy within the body to cope with the original pain rather than being dissipated in the anguish resulting from the pain.

These findings are the basis upon which the principles of acupuncture anaesthesia have been developed. At present the use of acupuncture anaesthesia has been confined mainly to Oriental countries, but since Richard Nixon's trip to China it has also been used in the United States. Its ever-growing popularity is due to the fact that it is highly successful in surgical procedures and has absolutely none of the negative side effects of the orthodox anaesthetics.

3

THE HISTORY OF ACUPUNCTURE

That in a situation overshadowed by strife, violence, and death would be born one of the noblest humanitarian sciences the world has ever known is indeed paradoxical. Nevertheless, in the dawn of history when stones and arrows were the only implements of war, many soldiers wounded on the battlefield reported that symptoms of disease that had plagued them for years had suddenly vanished. Naturally such strange occurrences baffled the physicians who could find no logical relationship between trauma and the ensuing recovery of health. Finally after many years of meticulous observation it was concluded that certain illnesses could actually be cured by striking or piercing specific points on the surface of the body. Of course the instruments of healing were modified from stones and arrows to fish bones, bamboo slips, and finally to needles made of gold, copper, and steel.

The *Nei Ching* or *The Yellow Emperor's Classic of Internal Medicine*, is the earliest known text on acupuncture. Believed to have been written during the reign of Emperor Huang Ti (2697–2596 B.C.), the *Nei Ching* elaborately outlines an all-inclusive, systematic method of therapy that also provided a foundation for all later developments in this science.

In the seventeenth century, Jesuit missionaries were sent to China so that they might introduce the basic doctrines of
14

Christianity to the Orient. While their labors amounted to less than what was hoped for, their failure was to the advantage of the West; for their unbelievable accounts of Chinese physicians curing illnesses by inserting needles into the surface of the skin marked the introduction of acupuncture to the West and implanted a desire in many Western physicians to learn more about this unusual method of therapy. Having no source from which to derive any applicable knowledge, Western physicians could at best only theorize as to the underlying causes for the spectacular results of such seemingly simple therapeutic measures.

In 1928, the French sinologist and diplomat, Souile de Morant returned to France after serving as Consul in China where, as a result of his close friendships with many Chinese physicians, he had become thoroughly acquainted with the principles of acupuncture. While in China he also acquired a fluency in speaking and reading Chinese that prompted him to undertake

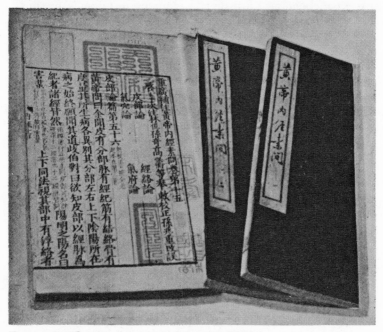

FIGURE 9. *The opening page of the* Nei Ching.

the task of translating the ancient Chinese manuscripts into French. Due to his arduous labors Western physicians were finally provided with a sound basis from which to study and apply this ancient science.

In 1884, Emperor Tao-Kuang in an imperial decree prohibited the practice of acupuncture within the imperial palace declaring that any physician who dared to touch the body of any member of the royal family was guilty of a serious transgression and subject to punishment. Consequently the scope of its practice was confined to the common people.

During the Long March of 1934–35, Mao Tse Tung's army, living and fighting under the most arduous conditions, used acupuncture almost exclusively and in lieu of any other form of medicine. The health of the army was maintained and serious illnesses and epidemics were avoided by the extensive use of this ancient science. This led Mao to conclude that acupuncture was a vital step toward the rebirth of a new China and it has once again become an essential element in China's medical system.

Japan established faculties of Western medicine at the university level during the latter part of the nineteenth century. Acupuncture, practiced by the Japanese since the sixth century, was abandoned there at the same time that it was officially proscribed in China by Emperor Tao-Kuang. But its efficacy in the treatment of disease kept it alive through the years until the present time when it has once again become the subject of intensive research at hospitals, medical centers, and universities.

At present acupuncture is practiced in Italy, Britain, West Germany, Argentina, and in several of the Socialist nations but France surpasses them all in that acupuncture is practiced there by approximately 6000 doctors and it is also a routine treatment in no less than 15 hospitals. Acupuncture has now become a focus of growing interest in the United States also. If the last 40 years are any indication of the future, it may someday be said that the latter part of the twentieth century saw the birth of the "Golden Age" of acupuncture.

4

THE IMPORTANCE OF THE ENERGY THEORY IN ACUPUNCTURE

*The root of the way of life, of birth and change is Qi
(energy); the myriad things of heaven and earth all
obey this law. Thus Qi in the periphery envelopes
heaven and earth, Qi in the interior activates them.
The source wherefrom the sun, moon, and stars
derive their light, the thunder, rain, wind and cloud
their being, the four seasons and the myriad things
their birth, growth, gathering and storing: all this is
brought about by Qi. Man's possession of life is
completely dependent upon this Qi.*   Nei Ching

The ancient Chinese texts expounding on the basic energy
supporting all life and matter in the cosmos were written to
convey basic scientific principles in a style that attracted the
attention even of those who were not inclined toward a serious
study of science. This is not to imply that the barriers between
the artistic, scientific, and practical ways of life were as distinct
and affecting such a marked degree of specialization as are
those characterizing modern civilization. The integrated man,
as he existed in ancient China, was one who constantly strived
to maintain a balance between the various life styles—the
artistic, the scientific, and the practical. It was no great effort
for the scientist to record his observations in a style which today
would be called poetic in form—it came to him naturally. That

17

scientific principles could be conveyed in such imaginative form attests to the unification of art and science typifying the golden age of Chinese civilization.

It may well be that because the basic principles of Chinese medical science are so poetically stated many modern scientists wish to reject them, avowing them to be "unscientific," "purely philosophical," "mystical," and "primitive." But the rejection of traditional principles on these grounds, far from indicating a greater degree of objective awareness on the part of modern day men of science, suggests instead a growing gap between science and a true "art of living." The principles of Chinese medical science as they have come down through the ages are just as applicable today as they were in the past, but they must be interpreted through a proper understanding of the poetic form that has enshrined and carried them through the ages.

THE NATURE OF ENERGY

Energy is a dynamic force in constant flux that circulates throughout the body. Many people plausibly substitute the word *life* for the word *energy* since the essential difference between the two words is so subtle that it eludes all but semanticists. Each term is vital to developing an accurate understanding of the energy theory as it applies to the body.

For all practical purposes, it can be stated that life is an *indication* of energy within the body. All that comes to mind on hearing the word *life*—breathing, talking, sleeping, eating, even the ability to read, think, and hear—all these can be achieved only because of the energy within the body. This invariably applies to those functions or activities that are not conspicuously perceptible: the metabolic processes within each single cell could not be accomplished without energy to sustain those functions. Energy is the basis for the apparent solid structures of the body also—all that pertains to its anatomy; for what is a solid structure such as a bone except a mass of living cells? All forms and activities of life, both anatomical and physiological, are supported by, and simultaneously deplete, the energy within the body.

Although most people assume that inert matter is completely solid or dense, it is energy that binds the protons, electrons, and neutrons within each individual atom. Inanimate matter, then, is simply energy at a different rate of vibration than that of other forms of life. *Energy therefore is the absolute basis for all forms of life and matter in the universe.*

Developing a comprehension of energy and all that pertains to a specific mode of its expression—in this case, the human body—enables a practitioner of acupuncture to cause the sensational, so-called "miracles" traditionally ascribed to this ancient science. Being thoroughly acquainted with the precise manner in which energy exists within the body, an experienced practitioner can beneficently manipulate this most subtle, all-pervading force. Since energy supports all vital functions associated with the body, the ability to adjust that energy enables one to regulate those functions which that energy supports; in an identical manner, dysfunctions (disease) of the body are eliminated by readjusting the energy imbalance that is the unseen cause of the apparent dysfunction. A person placidly undergoing major surgery and remaining fully conscious while under the influence of acupunctural anaesthesia is a perfect example of what an understanding of energy, and how it enlivens the body, enables a practitioner to do.

Food and air are considered to be the primary sources of energy depleted through daily living rather than fuel to be metabolized by the body. Energy, though, is not obtained from the gross molecular aspects of food and air, but rather from what can be called its "vibrational" essence, or, its electromagnetism. For instance: the nutrients within any particular food can be accurately reproduced in a biochemist's laboratory but life cannot be sustained over a prolonged period of time by ingesting those synthetic nutrients alone; it is possible to obtain every single vitamin, mineral, and chemical that comprise an egg, yet it is impossible to transform them into anything that vaguely resembles a genuine egg; neither is a person able to exist over a prolonged period of time on pure oxygen that has been obtained by laboratory methods, or in a room in which the air has been filtered by an electrical air-conditioner. In all of these instances something is lacking, and that "something" is the particular object's *life* essence—its electro-magnetism—that invisible energy that enlivens the gross molecular aspects of any object.

Electro-magnetism is a force with which most of us are not yet familiar. It was Western scientists who ingeniously verified the existence of electro-magnetism, providing a means for the logical explanation of many of the previously unexplainable phenomena resulting from acupuncture therapy. In short, electro-magnetism is a high intensity force that permeates the atomic and molecular structures of all objects including the surrounding atmosphere; because it is a natural force, it has a rapport with the energy within the body. When needles are inserted into the skin they act as antennae that conduct the electro-magnetic energy from the air into the body; therefore, electro-magnetic energy can replenish the body's energy that has been depleted through daily living.

THE MERIDIANS

Energy circulates throughout the body along minute pathways called *meridians*. An understanding of the meridians and their vital function of providing every cell of the body with energy is mandatory to the ultimate development of an unassailable expertise in administering therapy, for it is stated in the ancient texts:

> The means whereby man is created, the means whereby diseases occur, the means whereby man is cured, the means whereby disease arises: the twelve meridians are the basis for all theory and treatment.
> *(Nei Ching)*

and,

The meridian is that which decides over life and death. Through it the hundred diseases may be treated. *(Nei Ching)*

Regarding the meridians, Dr. Kim Bong Han of the University of Pyongang in North Korea, after conducting an extensive series of experiments, arrived at a conclusion for the actual existence of these pathways for energy. He reported that the meridians were actually composed of a type of histological tissue as yet unnoticed by scientists who, prior to Dr. Kim's experiments, had believed that the meridians were simply *imaginary* lines. He discovered the structure and function of the meridian system to be totally different from that of the lymphatic, circulatory, and nervous systems.

The meridians are channels (diameter 20-50 millimicrons) that are symmetrical and bilateral which exist beneath the surface of the skin; they have a thin membranous wall and are filled with a transparent, colorless fluid. Each of the main meridians intricately develops subsidiary branches, some of which supply adjacent areas with energy while others ultimately reach the surface of the skin. The places at which the branches reach the skin's surface are designated the points as illustrated on an acupuncture chart. Often several branches from different main channels converge at a single point; by stimulating that point, the energy in several channels can be affected simultaneously. The meridians are encircled by blood vessels that are especially in abundance around the individual branches that stem from each of the main channels. The phenomenon of bleeding that some patients report after undergoing acupuncture is an indication that the practitioner has narrowly missed the point on the surface of the skin and pierced one or many of the vascular vessels surrounding the point.

After conducting a series of experiments, German scientists discovered that the meridians are pathways for electricity. This led to the invention of a machine called the Point-locator which indicates the points where the branches of the meridians reach the skin's surface. At present the quality of the impulse that travels along the meridians is the subject of intensive research among Chinese scientists while many Western investigators are currently trying to determine possible associations between the meridians and the autonomic nervous system.

The meridian system, in being a physiological structure, provides a means by which many of the energy principles that have been labeled as purely hypothetical—even to the point where their actual existence is questioned—can be proved valid. For since the reality of the meridian system was experimentally verified by researchers like Dr. Kim, we can now conclude that the main functional purpose for which that system exists is to provide an effective means of expression for that all-pervading but invisible energy that animates all manifestations of life. Their delicate subtlety, when perceived in relationship to even the most microscopic aspects of the gross physical body, suggests that the meridians may well be the "missing-link," or the threshold, between pure energy and its first manifestation as microscopic matter.

Meridian is a word borrowed from geography indicating a thin line joining a series of ordered points. There are 12 main meridians—one assigned to each of the five organs, the six bowels, and the pericardium (here referred to as the heart constrictor). (The idea of six bowels is often perplexing to those unacquainted with acupuncture philosophy. In Chinese medicine the term "bowels" encompasses a much broader concept than that which most people attribute to it. The bowels are explained in detail in a following section.)

Although the first scientific proof of the existence of the meridian system is believed to be the result of Dr. Kim's efforts, conclusive evidence for the existence of the meridians was actually found in 1937 by Sir Thomas Lewis of England. His report, published in the *British Medical Journal* of February 1937, stated that he had discovered an "unknown nervous system" that was unrelated to either the sensory or the sympathetic nervous systems. Rather than being composed of a network of nerves, he reported, his newly discovered system was composed of a network of thin lines. Although his report went relatively unnoticed by his colleagues, it was the first concrete verification of a physiological system that Chinese medicine theoretically claimed to exist thousands of years ago.

THE POINTS OF ENTRY AND EXIT

Each of the main meridians has both a point of entry and a point of exit. Energy enters the meridian at the point of entry, circulates along the meridian, and flows through the point of exit on through the point of entry of the succeeding meridian. The point of exit on a meridian is connected to the point of entry on the succeeding meridian by a secondary channel. Treating a point of entry will affect the entire length of the meridian in that the direction of the flow of energy along a meridian remains constant and never vacillates after flowing through the point of entry. Figure 22 illustrates the points of entry and exit.

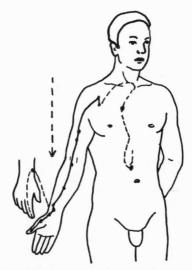

FIGURE 10. *This is the Lung Meridian with a descending flow of energy running from the top of the chest, along the inside of the arm to the outside of the thumb; it joins a series of 11 bilateral points.*

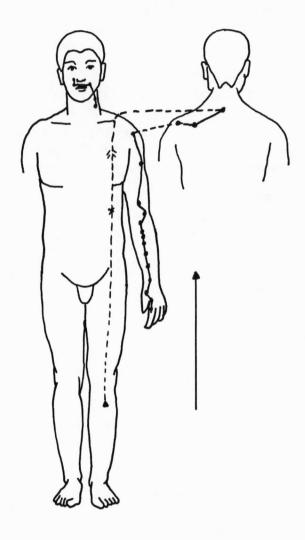

FIGURE 11. *This is the Large Intestine Meridian with an ascending flow of energy running from the tip of the index finger of the hand to the base of the eye; it joins a series of 20 bilateral points.*

24

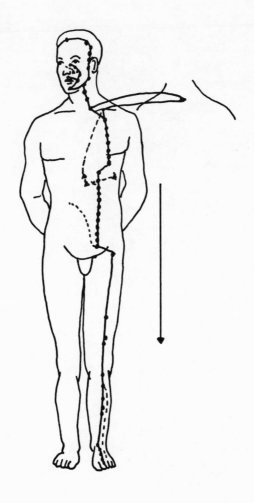

FIGURE 12. *This is the Stomach Meridian with a descending flow of energy running from the head to the foot; it joins a series of 45 bilateral points.*

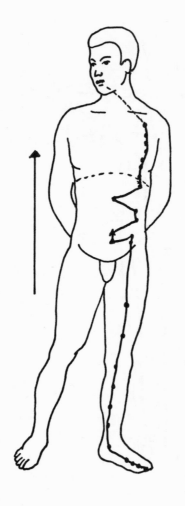

FIGURE 13. *This is the Spleen-Pancreas Meridian with
an ascending flow of energy running from the foot to
the chest; it joins a series of 21 bilateral points.*

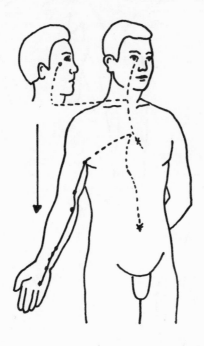

FIGURE 14. *This is the Heart Meridian with a descending flow of energy running from the chest to the hand; it joins a series of 9 bilateral points.*

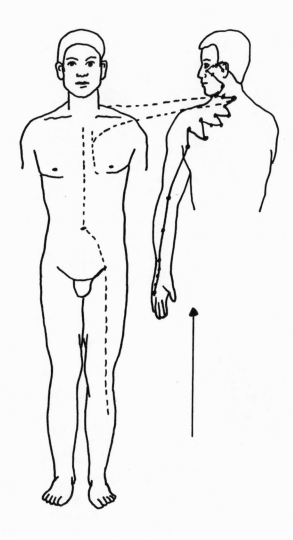

FIGURE 15. *This is the Small Intestine Meridian with an ascending flow of energy running from the hand to the head; it joins a series of 19 points.*

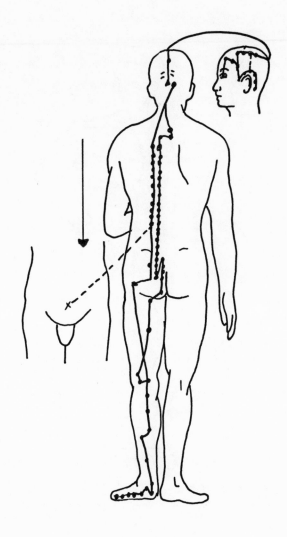

FIGURE 16. *This is the Bladder Meridian with a descending flow of energy running from the head to the foot; it joins a series of 67 bilateral points.*

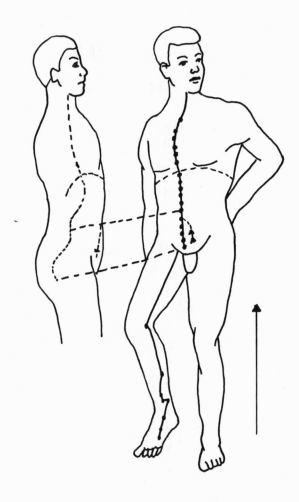

FIGURE 17. *This is the Kidney Meridian with an ascending flow of energy running from the foot to the chest; it joins a series of 27 bilateral points.*

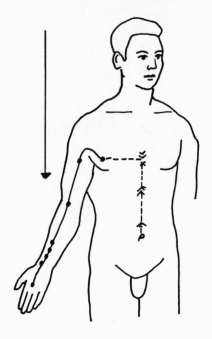

FIGURE 18. *This is the Heart Constrictor Meridian with a descending flow of energy running from the chest to the hand; it joins a series of 9 bilateral points.*

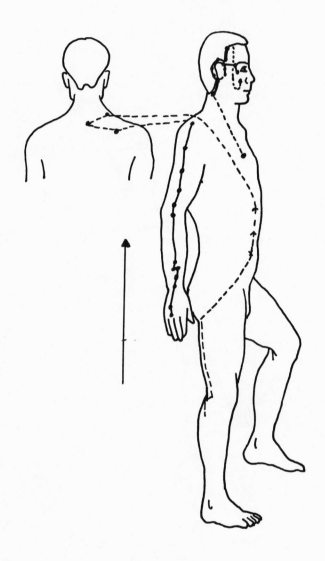

FIGURE 19. *This is the Triple Heater Meridian with an ascending flow of energy running from the hand to the head; it joins a series of 23 bilateral points.*

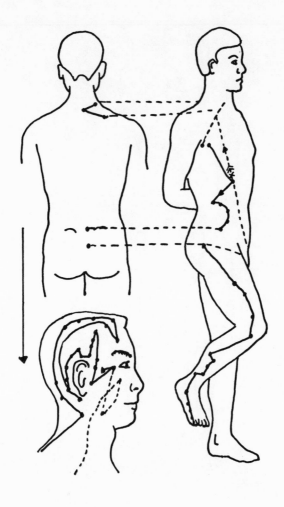

FIGURE 20. *This is the Gallbladder Meridian with a descending flow of energy running from the chest to the foot; it joins a series of 44 bilateral points.*

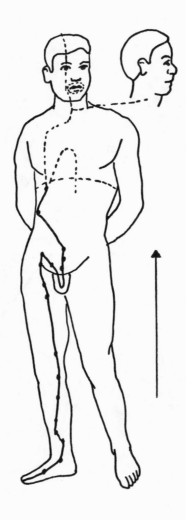

FIGURE 21. *This is the Liver Meridian with an ascending flow of energy running from the foot to the chest; it joins a series of 14 bilateral points.*

34

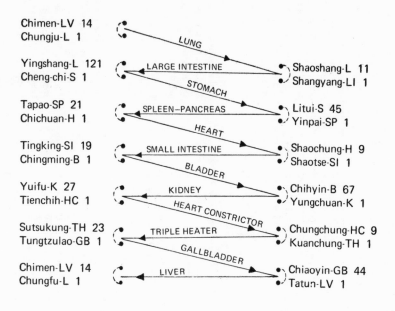

Chimen-LV 14
Chungju-L 1

LUNG

Yingshang-L 121
Cheng-chi-S 1

LARGE INTESTINE

Shaoshang-L 11
Shangyang-LI 1

STOMACH

Tapao-SP 21
Chichuan-H 1

SPLEEN–PANCREAS

Litui-S 45
Yinpai-SP 1

HEART

Tingking-SI 19
Chingming-B 1

SMALL INTESTINE

Shaochung-H 9
Shaotse-SI 1

BLADDER

Yuifu-K 27
Tienchih-HC 1

KIDNEY

Chihyin-B 67
Yungchuan-K 1

HEART CONSTRICTOR

Sutsukung-TH 23
Tungtzulao-GB 1

TRIPLE HEATER

Chungchung-HC 9
Kuanchung-TH 1

GALLBLADDER

Chimen-LV 14
Chungfu-L 1

LIVER

Chiaoyin-GB 44
Tatun-LV 1

FIGURE 22. *Sequence of energy flow illustrating the points of entry and exit.*

TABLE 1. *The Circulation and Distribution of the Twelve Meridians and Their Main Treatments.*

Meridian	Circulating Pathway	Relating Organs	Main Treatment
Arm Greater Yin (Lung)	Leaving the subscapular area this runs along the anterior part of the upper arm along the outer side of the anterior surface of the forearm and ends at a point in the thumb.	Belongs to the lung. Communicated with the large intestine and is connected with the stomach.	Diseases of the thorax, lung, trachea and pharynx-larynx, etc.
Arm Absolute Yin (Circulation-sex)	This arises in the chest just below the diaphragm. It emerges at the side of the nipple and then descends down the upper limb between the meridians of the heart and the lung and ends at the middle finger.	Belongs to the Heart Constrictor and is communicated with the triple heater.	Diseases of the heart, thorax, stomach and nervous system.
Arm Lesser Yin (Heart)	Starts in the hollow of the armpit and then runs down the inside of the anterior surface of the arm to end in the little finger.	Belongs to the heart, is communicated with the small intestine and is connected with the inner pharynx and the tissue behind the eyeball (the eye system).	Diseases of the heart, thorax and nervous system.

The Three Arm Yang Meridians

	Pathway	Organ relationship	Diseases treated
Arm Sunlight Yang (Large Intestine)	Commencing at the extremity of the index finger it extends along the outer border of the arm and shoulder, along the lateral side of the neck and ends near the nose.	Belongs to the large intestine and is communicated with the lung.	Diseases of the ear, nose, pharynx, tooth, head and neck.
Arm Lesser Yang (Triple Heater)	Starts at the tip of the ring finger, runs up the arm between the meridians of the large intestine and small intestine passing along the back of the shoulderblade, turns round the ear to the temple and ends near the outside of the eyebrow.	Belongs to the triple heater and is communicated with the circulation-sex and distributed in the thoracic cavity between the breasts.	Diseases of the ear, heart and thoracic region.
Arm Greater Yang (Small Intestine)	Originates at the end of the little finger and runs along the inside of the posterior surface of the arm, passes behind the shoulder and shoulderblade across the neck to end in front of the ear.	Belongs to the small intestine and is communicated with the heart, and is connected with the esophagus and stomach.	Deaf-mutism and diseases of the head, face, five senses, neck and shoulder region.

The Three Arm Yin Meridians

37

The Three Leg Yang Meridians			
Leg Sunlight Yang (Stomach)	Beginning on the face it descends along the front of the thorax and follows the outer and front side of the leg to end in the second toe.	Belongs to the stomach, is communicated with the spleen.	Diseases of the head, face, eye, ear, tooth, pharynx-larynx, stomach and intestine.
Leg Lesser Yang (Gallbladder)	Starts at the outer canthus of the eye, runs over the head to the mastoid, returns again to the front of the ear and then passes to the back of the head past the neck and shoulder to the armpit along the side of the chest to the neighborhood of the hip joint and down the outside of the leg to end at the fourth toe.	Belongs to the gallbladder, is communicated with the liver.	Diseases of the temporal region, flank of the chest region and limbs.
Leg Greater Yang (Bladder)	Starts at the inner canthus of the eye, it winds round the head and neck following the spinal column and reaching the coccyx. It ascends to the outside of the shoulderblade and it redescends parallel to its original course down the back of the leg and ends in the fifth toe.	Belongs to the bladder, is communicated with the kidney and is connected with the brain.	Diseases of the head, nape, eye, nose, lumbar region and the internal organ which is connected with the "Shu point" of this meridian.

The Three Leg Yin Meridians			
Leg Greater Yin (Spleen)	Commencing on the tip of the big toe, this meridian follows a course along the outer and inner side of the leg, then along the body midway between nipple and axillary line to end in the outside of the thorax.	Belongs to the spleen, is communicated with the stomach and is connected with the heart and tongue.	Diseases of the gastro-intestinal tract and the urinary and reproductive system.
Leg Absolute Yin (Liver)	Commencing at the outside of the big toe, this meridian runs along the inside of the leg, up the trunk and ends at the costal margin near the nipple.	Belongs to the liver, is communicated with the gallbladder and is connected with the stomach, lung, pharynx and larynx, jaws and the tissue behind the eyeball.	Diseases of the urinary and reproductive system, liver and gallbladder.
Leg Lesser Yin (Kidney)	Starts under the little toe ascends the inside of the leg and thigh and courses along the front of the ear to end near the clavicle.	Belongs to the kidney, is communicated with the bladder and is connected with the liver, lung, heart, inside of the thoracic cavity and of the tongue.	Diseases of the urinary and reproductive system.

The meridians are the means by which the organs and bowels are linked together and by which each organ and bowel is enlivened by energy as it circulates along the meridian circuit. A question that might naturally arise as a result of the preceding illustrations depicting the sequence of the main meridians is, "If an organ or bowel associated with one of the main meridians were to become diseased, according to the information given thus far, wouldn't it be logical to conclude that the energy would be blocked and unable to complete its cycle of circulation?" No, because in addition to the twelve main meridians there are eight extraordinary meridians that provide for the circulation of energy when it becomes superfluous or excessive in one of the main meridians.

THE EIGHT EXTRAORDINARY MERIDIANS

The eight extraordinary meridians can justifiably be called "life-savers" in that they provide for energy to continue its cycle of circulation regardless of whether any one of the organs or bowels becomes diseased and blocks the meridian circuit. Traditional Chinese medicine explains the purpose of the eight extraordinary meridians in an analogous manner by likening them to drainage ditches and dykes that would exist alongside a major river which, of course, corresponds to the main or major meridians. If for any reason the river (main meridian) should become flooded and overflow its banks, the drainage ditches will accommodate the superfluous water (energy). Therefore the flow of energy along the eight extraordinary meridians is not constant but is determined by the amount of excess energy in a main meridian.

Of the eight extraordinary meridians only two have acupuncture points of their own; the other six utilize points along the main meridians which they traverse. The two extraordinary meridians which have their own points are:

1) Jen-Mo Meridian, or the meridian of conception, has 24 single points with an ascending flow of energy running from the perineum to the chin;

2) Tu-Mo, or the governor meridian, has 27 single points with an ascending flow of energy running from the coccyx up along the back and atop the head ending at the upper gum.

Jen-Mo and Tu-Mo exist outside the general energy circulatory system and are related to it as secondary channels. The following figures illustrate the paths of the eight extraordinary meridians.

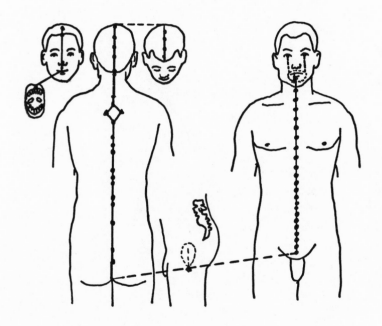

FIGURE 23. *Circulation of Tu-Mo and Jen-Mo.*

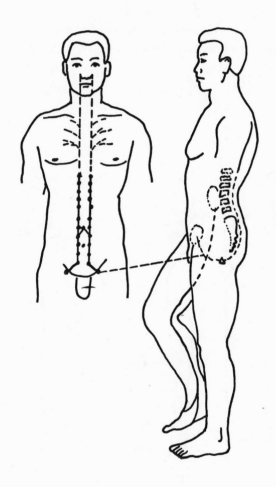

FIGURE 24. *Circulation of Chungmo.*

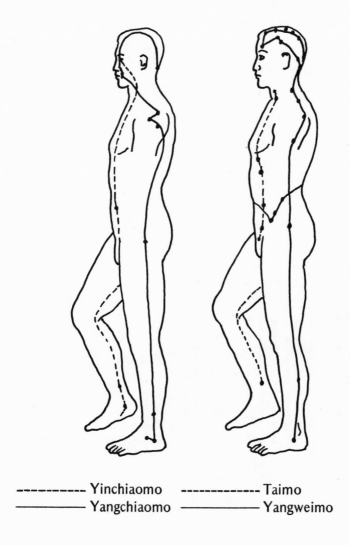

```
----------- Yinchiaomo    ------------- Taimo
——————— Yangchiaomo   ——————— Yangweimo
```

FIGURE 25. *Circulation of Yinchiaomo, Yangchiaomo, Yinweimo, Yangweimo, Taimo.*

TABLE 2. *Distribution, Relating Organs and 12 Main Meridians of the Eight Extra Meridians.*

Name	Pathway	Relating Organs	Function
Tu-Mo (Governing Vessel)	Starts at the perineum, up along the midst of the back to the vertex, down along the nose and ends in the gum of the upper lip.	Kidneys, uterus, spinal cord, brain.	Related with Arm and Leg Yang meridians (the governor of Yang). Connected with Leg Greater Yang meridian on point Houhsi.
Jen-Mo (Vessel of Conception)	Starts at the perineum up along the midst of the abdomen and chest, runs to the chin, winds round the lips and ends below the eye.	Uterus, eyes.	Related with Arm and Leg Yin meridians (sea of Yin), connected with Arm Greater Yin meridian on Liehchueh point.
Chungmo	1. Originates from the perineum, runs along the femoral sulcus up together with Leg Lesser Yin meridian, passing the abdomen and chest, joins with Jen-Mo, winds round the lips, enters the palate and ends below the eye. 2. From the femoral sulcus along the inside of the lower limb to the posterior side of the internal malleolus and basis of the foot; a branch starting from the internal malleolus runs to the dorsal part of the foot. 3. Together with Tu-Mo circulate on the back along the spinal column.	Uterus, spinal cord, kidneys, eyes.	Related with Jen-Mo, Tu-Mo, Leg Sunlight Yang meridian, Leg Lesser Yin meridian, is the sea of the 12 meridians, also called "sea of blood." Chungmo is connected with Leg Greater Yin meridian on Kungsun point.

44

Name	Course	Related organs	Relations
Taimo	Originates from below the 2nd lumbar vertebra, winds round the loins and abdomen.		Related with each of the straight forwarding meridians on the lumbar and abdominal region, has a restraining effect on the meridians, is connected with Leg Lesser Yang meridian on Linchi point.
Yangchiaomo	Starts from the external malleolus, runs along the outside of the lower limb, is distributed on the flank, winds round the shoulder, runs to the corner of the mouth and reaches the medial angle of the eye, then together with Yinchiaomo ascends to the posterior side of the auricle, entering into the brain.	Ear, eye, brain.	Related with the three Yang meridians of the leg, Arm Greater Yang meridian, Arm Sunlight Yang meridian and Tu-Mo govern the Yang meridians on both sides of the body and are connected with Leg Greater Yang meridian on Shenmo point.
Yinchiaomo	Starts from the internal malleolus, runs along the inside of the lower limb, passing the Yin organs and chest, runs to the throat and reaches the medial angle of the eye; together with Yangchiaomo ascends to the posterior side of the auricle entering into the brain.	Ear, eye, brain, pharynx and larynx.	Related with Leg Lesser Yin meridian, Leg Greater Yin meridian and Jen-Mo, governs the Yin meridians on both sides of the body, is connected with Leg Lesser Yin meridian on Chaohai point.

Yangweimo	The Mochi originates from the Yang meridians, from the knee runs along the outside of the abdomen and chest, reaches the shoulder, upwards to the posterior side of the auricle and ends on the vertex, and joins with Tu-Mo.	Ear	Related with the Yang meridians of the Arm and Leg and with Tu-Mo, governs the outside of the body and is connected with Arm Lesser Yang meridian on Waikuan point.
Yinweimo	The Mochi originates from the Yin meridians, from the inside of the knee runs along the abdomen and chest, ends in pharynx and larynx, and joins with Jen-Mo.	Each Tsang Fu in the thoracic and abdominal cavity.	Related with the three Yin meridians of the Leg and Jen-Mo. Governs the inside of the body, is connected with Arm Absolute Yin meridian on Neikuan point.

On many occasions after I've presented a lecture on the energy theory and the meridians, people will approach me and say, "Why, I never realized how greatly the nerves control the body!" or, "I understood your lecture because when I was in college I took an anatomy course and the professor spent an unusually long time on the nervous system." I must emphasize that the nervous system and the meridian system are totally different from one another! Although many researchers and physicians have attributed the efficacy of acupuncture to the functioning of the nervous system, it must be understood that the nervous system, as subtle as it may be, is still grosser than the meridian system. Without the meridians supplying every part of the body—including the individual neurons (nerve cells)—with energy, the nerves would simply be a mass of lifeless fibers; the energy flowing along the meridians actually enlivens the most microscopic nerve fibers enabling them to perform their function—that is, to transmit impulses from the external or internal environment.

The existence of electro-magnetic energy was unquestionably demonstrated to me as a result of a fatal disease that suddenly afflicted a number of my prize gardenias—a most fragrant flower that my family has cultivated for generations with great pride. I was perplexed when the flowers began to develop a blackish, coal-like hue and the leaves began to droop and wither. All my efforts to save the gardenias were of no avail and within three days the disease appeared to have killed the plants. It suddenly dawned on me that I should try acupuncture on the plants. After all, the plants were apparently dead and although my decision to try acupuncture seemed outlandish (for the sole reason that I had no idea as to the localization of treatment points on a plant) any effort was better than no effort at all. I inserted needles into the stems and leaves at places where I had deduced that points should exist and let the needles remain intact for approximately 20 to 30 minutes. After two days of treatments I noticed a faint green pigment beginning to appear around the points I had treated. On the third day it was quite obvious that the plants would recover; they had almost totally regained their natural pigment and their previously wilted leaves once again automatically turned in the direction of the life-giving rays of the sun.

THE AROUND-THE-WORLD MASSAGE

Having completed this introduction to the energy theory and the meridians, I would like to offer you a method of massage that will be absolutely invaluable in that it will augment the energy within the body, provide for a constant and unimpeded flow of energy along the meridians, and will eventually rejuvenate not only an aging body but a fatigued mind as well. I have very appropriately named this invigorating massage the "Around-the-World Massage" for it stimulates the energy along all of the main meridians thereby concurrently affecting the"energy in all areas adjacent to those meridians. Applying the following technique will enable you to become simultaneously acquainted with both the paths of the main meridians—an absolute necessity for aspiring practitioners, and also to intimately experience the exhilarating effects of such a simple method of massage.

Using the bulb of the thumb or of the index and middle fingers, gently massage the entire length of each of the main meridians *in the direction of the flow of energy* along the meridian (chapter 1, figure 4). It is advised that the meridians be massaged in the prescribed sequence as they are illustrated in figures 10 thru 21 and not in any haphazard, random order. The reason for this should be obvious, for the purpose of meridian massage is to stimulate and "build" an unbroken circle of energy circulating within the body and this can only be accomplished by massaging the meridians in the prescribed sequence. Baby oil, massage lotions, ginger juice, etc., may be used to lubricate the surface of the skin.

MERIDIAN MEDITATION

After becoming thoroughly acquainted with the paths of the twelve main meridians and with the flow of energy within the body as a result of the preceding meridian massage, one may commence the following method entitled "Meridian Meditation." Meridian meditation is a method for both physical and spiritual development that is a standard practice elaborately described in the philosophy of Taoism of which acupuncture itself is one of the various branches. The venerated sage and philosopher, Lao-Tzu purportedly lived anywhere from 160 to 500 years and faithfully practiced, and strongly advocated the practice of, meridian meditation to his disciples.

The method of meridian meditation consists of first finding a comfortable position. Sitting on a soft cushion is preferable; keep the spinal column erect but not rigid and the shoulders will automatically fall into their natural position. Next empty the mind of all irrelevant, excess thoughts and focus all of your attention upon the lung meridian. Trace the path of the lung meridian with your index and middle finger paying close attention to the concurrent subjective feelings that arise as a result of this procedure. Mentally follow the flow of energy as it descends along the lung meridian and then repeat the same procedure along the large intestine meridian which has an ascending flow of energy. Massaging the entire length of all twelve of the main meridians will eventually enable one to sense the most minute energy fluctuation along the meridian circuit. Ultimately one will be able to willfully direct the energy flow along any one of the meridians. Becoming consciously aware of the circulation of energy within the body will confer longevity of life, for this ability will enable one to maintain a state of energy balance under any and all circumstances. Disease can only inhabit a body in which there is an erratic flow of energy along the meridians.

THE ORGANS AND BOWELS

Chinese medicine lists the five organs inside the body as: the heart, spleen-pancreas, lungs, kidneys, and liver; and lists the six bowels as: the large intestine, bladder, triple heater, gallbladder, small intestine, and stomach. Another part of the body, the heart constrictor or pericardium, corresponds to the blood vessel system. Classification of each of the viscera as either an organ or a bowel is determined by its physiological structure and function. Chinese medicine designates the five organs as *Tsang* (solid); the six bowels are *Fu* (hollow).

> What are called the five solid organs store life essence and energy and do not let them leak away; therefore they are filled but cannot be full. The six hollow bowels transmit and transform food but do not store it; thus they are full but cannot be filled.
> *(Nei Ching)*

The distinguishing characteristic of an organ is that it is a solid structure that has predominantly an internal function—it "stores but does not transmit." The distinguishing characteristic of a bowel is that it is a hollow structure and its functioning is primarily influenced by things outside the body—it "transforms food but does not retain." When referring to any one of the organs or bowels, and the heart constrictor, the Chinese not only include all aspects of its apparent physiological structure, but also all that pertains to its imperceptible function; in Chinese medicine, structure and function are synonymous. The organ of the heart includes its obvious organic structure and rhythmical beating in addition to its function of circulating blood throughout the body. The bowel of the large intestine includes both its apparent physiological structure and its function which is the final evanescent absorption of nutrients from the digested food as it moves along the intestinal tract.

The organs are *Yin* in that their functions are predominantly *internal*. The bowels are *Yang* in that their primary functions are influenced by things *outside* the body. The concept of Yin and Yang is elaborated upon in greater detail in Chapter 5. For the moment it will suffice to state that Yin and Yang are complementary and opposite. In order to maintain a perfect balance within the body, each Yin organ has a complementary Yang bowel; if the functioning of an organ or bowel is not relative to its complementary organ or bowel, the flow of energy throughout the body will be impeded. Therefore the perfect balance of Yin and Yang (organ and bowel) is crucial.

Five organs, six bowels, and one heart constrictor amount to a total of 12 which correlates precisely to the 12 main meridians of the body. As illustrated in the beginning of this chapter, the manner in which the meridians are interconnected is suggestive of an unbroken circle which provides for the perpetual circulation of energy throughout the body. As the energy flows along the meridians, each of the organs, and bowels, and the heart constrictor is provided with its quantum of vital force for maintaining the life-sustaining functions. When referring to an individual organ or bowel, Chinese medicine does not imply that it be perceived as being distinctly separate or as existing apart from the other viscera, but suggests that instead each be viewed as one segment of a wheel or circle, with each segment being equally important to the harmonious functioning of the whole. The perfect functioning of each of the organs, bowels, and heart constrictor is considered basic to maintaining an overall state of perfect balance within the body.

THE FIVE ELEMENTS AND THEIR CYCLES OF INTERACTION

Energy flows through the body via the meridians and their respective organs and bowels in well-defined cycles; the cycles depicting the flow of energy within the body are an exact reflection of the cyclic energy interaction between the five earthly elements. The five earthly elements are: fire, earth, metal, water, and wood; there are two cycles that illustrate the interaction between these elements. In the first cycle—the cycle of generation—each element *generates,* or *produces* the succeeding element: thus fire produces earth, earth produces metal, metal produces water, water produces wood, wood produces fire, fire produces earth—the cycle begins again. In the second cycle—the cycle of destruction—each element *destroys* or *absorbs* the succeeding element: thus fire destroys metal, metal destroys wood, wood absorbs water, water absorbs fire, fire destroys metal—the cycle begins again.

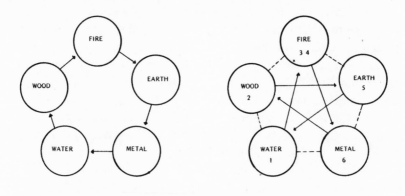

FIGURE 26.   FIGURE 27.

The importance of the two preceding cycles is in that they form the basis for the application of acupuncture therapy. In affirming man to be the microcosm—the reflection of the macrocosm—the Chinese believe that the interaction of his bodily functions mirror the two preceding cycles that depict the interaction between the five earthly elements. Chinese medicine identifies each of the viscera with one of the elements in the following manner:

fire—heart
    small intestine
    triple heater
    heart constrictor
earth—spleen-pancreas
    stomach

metal—lungs
    large intestine
water—kidneys
    bladder
wood—liver
    gallbladder

The elements as assigned to the Organs and Bowels are:

TABLE 3.

	Wood	Fire (Prince)	Earth	Metal	Water	Fire (Minister)
TSANG— Organ	Liver	Heart	Spleen	Lungs	Kidneys	Heart Constrictor
FU— Bowel	Gallbladder	Small Intestine	Stomach	Large Intestine	Bladder	Triple Heater

Identifying each of the organs with its respective element in the first cycle results in: the heart (fire) supporting the spleen-pancreas (earth); the spleen-pancreas (earth), the lungs (metal); the lungs (metal), the kidneys (water); the kidneys (water), the liver (wood); the liver (wood), the heart (fire). The bowels also follow the same cycle: the small intestine (fire) supports the stomach (earth); the stomach (earth), the large intestine (metal); the large intestine (metal) the bladder (water); the bladder (water), the gallbladder (wood).

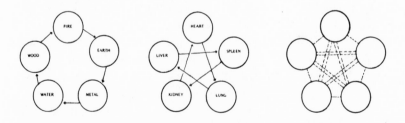

FIGURE 28.

If the energy within an organ is not balanced, that organ, rather than being able to effectively support the organ succeeding it on the meridian circuit, will adversely affect, or will be adversely affected by, another organ; this pattern has been depicted in the second cycle of the interaction between the elements in which each element destroys or absorbs the other. Thus, when the energy within the heart (fire) is imbalanced, it (heart, fire) will adversely affect the lungs (metal); the lungs (metal), the liver (wood); the liver (wood), the spleen-pancreas (earth); the spleen-pancreas (earth), the kidneys (water); the kidneys (water), the heart (fire). The second also applies to the bowels: imbalanced energy within the small intestine (fire) will cause it to adversely affect the large intestine (metal); the large intestine (metal), the gallbladder (wood); the gallbladder (wood), the stomach (earth); the stomach (earth), the bladder (water), the bladder (water), the small intestine (fire).

In discovering that the cyclic interaction between the organs and bowels is identical to the interaction between the elements, the ancient Chinese not only provided a means by which the sayings, "That which is above is the same as that which is below," and "The microcosm reflects the macrocosm" can be realized and understood, but they also provided a means whereby the interaction of energy between the organs and bowels can be accepted as fact in that the basis for that interaction is founded upon the very same logic whereby the interaction of the five earthly elements is instinctively realized to be true.

The following cases show how acupuncture is applied using the two basic cycles of interaction as a foundation for therapy. According to the Law of the Five Elements, the lungs (metal) support the kidneys (water). If the lungs are indisposed and consequently must utilize all of their energy to sustain their functions, the kidneys must necessarily become polluted as a result of not having an adequate amount of energy with which to function. To revitalize the kidneys it will be necessary to treat the lungs, thereby enabling them to support the kidneys. On the other hand it is also possible that the liver (wood), succeeding the kidneys on the meridian circuit, may require additional energy owing to a dysfunction, and obtaining that energy from the kidneys it thereby debilitates them. In this instance, treating the liver (wood) will automatically effect a cure within the kidneys (water).

If a person consumes large quantities of alcohol, the ensuing energy imbalance within the overworked kidneys will adver-

TABLE 4. *The Five Elements.*

ELEMENT	WOOD	FIRE	EARTH	METAL	WATER
Planet	Jupiter	Mars	Saturn	Venus	Mercury
Direction	East	South	Center	West	North
Season	Spring	Summer	Indian Summer	Autumn	Winter
Color	Blue	Red	Yellow	White	Black
Perverse Climates	Wind	Heat	Moisture	Dryness	Cold
Organ	Liver	Heart	Spleen	Lungs	Kidneys
Sense	Sight	Speech	Taste	Smell	Hearing
Parts of body	Muscles Nails	Pulse Complexion	Flesh Lips	Skin Body Hair	Bones Hair
Orifice	Eyes	Ears	Mouth	Nose	Anus Urinary
Fluid	Tears	Sweat	Lymph	Mucus	Saliva
Smell	Rancid	Burnt	Sweet	Fleshy	Putrid
Taste	Acid	Bitter	Sweet	Piquant	Salty
Sound	Cry	Laugh	Song	Sob	Groan
Psychic Values	Spirit	Conscience	Ideas	Animal Spirits	Will Ambition
Emotions	Anger	Joy	Worry	Grief	Fear
Dynamic Energy	Blood	Psychic Energy	Physical Energy	Vital Energy	Willpower
Governs	Lungs	Kidneys	Liver	Heart	Spleen
Social Estate	The People	The State	A Prince	A Vassal	What is produced
Animal (domestic)	Chicken	Dog	Ox	Horse	Pig
Animal (wild)	Tiger	Stag	Bear	Bird	Monkey
Grain	Wheat	Millet	Rye	Rice	Peas
Strain	Over-use of Eyes	Over Walking	Over Sitting	Over Lying Down	Over Standing

sely affect the heart. The energy imbalance within the kidneys will also disable them from supporting the liver that in turn must support the heart. In addition to not being supported by the kidneys, the liver must cope with the stress imposed upon it by the alcohol. Alcoholism and cardiac conditions go "hand-in-hand." With alcoholism, the energy within the kidneys, liver, and heart must be augmented simultaneously. The energy within the heart must be augmented so that organ will not draw energy from the liver; the energy of the liver will have to be augmented so it does not obtain its energy from the exhausted kidneys; and finally the energy within the kidneys must be balanced to neutralize it so it does not adversely affect the heart.

THE BASIC ORGAN/BOWEL UNITS

As stated previously, the organs are Yin and the bowels are Yang. Yin and Yang are opposite but neither can exist in total isolation from the other; they are opposites in the sense that they represent the different sides of the same coin. In the same manner, each Yin organ has a complementary Yang bowel; together they form a unit of which the perfect functioning of each organ or bowel is indispensable to the perfect functioning of the other. For example, the Yin organ of the lungs exists in relation to the Yang bowel of the large intestine. A perfect functioning of the lungs is necessary to provide an unimpeded flow of energy to the large intestine, for, as can be seen in the illustration of the order of the organs and bowels on the meridian circuit, the large intestine follows, or is preceded by, the lungs. The following units comprised of both a Yin organ and a Yang bowel exhibit the same functional relationship as that exemplified by the preceding lungs/large intestine unit:

heart/small intestine(fire)
bladder/kidneys(water)
heart constrictor/triple heater(fire)

gallbladder/liver(wood)
lungs/large intestine(metal)
stomach/spleen-pancreas(earth)

TABLE 5. *The Order of Five Elements (Organs & Bowels).*

1	(WATER)	Kidneys–Bladder
2	(WOOD)	Liver–Gallbladder
3	(FIRE)	Heart–Small Intestine
4	(FIRE)	Heart Constrictor–Triple Heater
5	(EARTH)	Spleen-Stomach
6	(METAL)	Lungs–Large Intestine

THE CONJUNCTIVE CHANNELS

The meridians associated with the organ and bowel comprising each of the basic units are conjoined by the conjunctive, or connective channels; the primary function of the conjunctive channels is to enable energy to flow between the viscera comprising each unit thereby strengthening the relationship between their meridians. For example, energy flows from the lungs to the large intestine; the two meridians associated with these viscera are coupled by a conjunctive channel existing between L 7 on the lung meridian and LI 6 on the large intestine meridian; both points are in the wrist.

TABLE 6. *Distribution of the Fifteen Lomo (Conjunctive Channels).*

Name of Lomo (conjunctive channel)	Point of Separation	Running to Meridian	Area of Distribution
Separation of Arm Greater Yin	Liehchueh (L7)	Arm Sunlight Yang	Enters into the palm, runs off the wrist.
Separation of Arm Lesser Yin	Tungli (H5)	Arm Greater Yang	Along the original meridian enters into the heart, is related with the root of the tongue and ends in the tissue behind the eye ball.

Separation of Arm Absolute Yin	Neikuan (HC6)	Arm Lesser Yang	Along the original meridian and is related with heart constrictor.
Separation of Arm Sunlight Yang	Pienli (LI6)	Arm Greater Yin	Passing the forearm, cheek, teeth, enters into the ear.
Separation of Arm Greater Yang	Chihcheng (SI7)	Arm Lesser Yin	Runs along the elbow and is connected with the shoulder joint.
Separation of Arm Lesser Yang	Waikuan (TH5)	Arm Absolute Yin	Winds around the forearm and is poured into the chest.
Separation of Leg Greater Yin	Kungsun (SP4)	Leg Sunlight Yang	Enters into the intestine and stomach.
Separation of Leg Lesser Yin	Tachung (K4)	Leg Greater Yang	Runs along the original meridian up to heart constrictor, penetrating the loin and back.
Separation of Leg Absolute Yin	Likou (LV5)	Leg Lesser Yang	Runs along the leg to the testes and ends in the penis.
Separation of Leg Sunlight Yang	Fenglung (S40)	Leg Greater Yin	Runs along the outside of the tibia to the vertex and enters into the throat.
Separation of Leg Greater Yang	Feiyang (B58)	Leg Lesser Yin	
Separation of Leg Lesser Yang	Kuangming (GB37)	Leg Absolute Yin	Enters into the dorsal side of the foot.
Separation of the Vessel of Conception	Weiyi (JEN15)		Spreads in the abdomen.
Separation of the Governing Vessel	Changchiang (TU1)		Runs upward to the neck, is spread on the head and runs beside Leg Greater Yang meridian.
The Great Lo of the Spleen	Tapao (SP21)		Spreads on the side of the chest.

To apply therapy to the basic units, stimulating the first member of each unit will simultaneously affect the second member; this phenomenon is the basis upon which the principles which the ancient Chinese called the "mother-child" law are founded.

> The "mother-child" law:
> If a meridian is empty, stimulate its mother. If it is full, disperse the child. *(Nei Ching)*

The mother-child law, as it applies to the human body, is based upon the interaction between the five elements. Each element is the "mother" of the succeeding element and, at the same time, the "child" of the element that precedes it as shown on the cycle depicting the flow of energy throughout the elements. For instance, earth is the mother of metal and also the child of fire.

As energy circulates throughout the body, it passes through each organ and bowel in a well-defined cycle. Each organ or bowel is the "mother" of the organ or bowel succeeding it on the meridian circuit; and each organ is also the "child" of the organ or bowel preceding it on the meridian circuit; this phenomenon is based on the law of the five elements. For example, the lungs support the kidneys and therefore the lungs are said to be the "mother" of the kidneys. If the energy within the kidneys (child) is deficient, according to the mother-child law, by stimulating the energy within the lungs (mother), the kidneys will automatically receive an increase of energy. In addition to stimulating the lungs, the energy of the liver must also be augmented so that the liver (child of the kidneys) does not absorb the energy from the kidneys. If the energy within the kidneys receives the initial stimulus, that stimulus, in addition to augmenting the energy within the kidneys, will augment the energy within the liver; for in this instance, rather than being the "child," the kidneys are the mother of the liver (child). If, in the preceding example, the energy within the "mother" is dispersed rather than augmented, the energy within the "child" will be dispersed also.

THE CYCLE OF GENERATION (SUPPORT)

Mother	Child
1) lungs/large intestine (metal) supports	bladder/kidney (water)
2) bladder/kidney (water)	gallbladder/liver (wood)
3) gallbladder/liver (wood)	heart/small intestine
4) heart/small intestine heart constrictor/triple heater (fire)	heart constrictor/triple heater (fire) stomach/spleen-pancreas (earth)
5) stomach/spleen-pancreas (earth)	lungs/large intestine (metal)

The conjoint functioning between each organ and bowel comprising any of the basic units is dependent on each organ and bowel of the unit being balanced in relation to the other; this balance is achieved by neutralizing any other organ or bowel that will adversely affect either member of the basic unit.

The functional relationship between the basic units as shown in the above cycle of generation is based upon the same cycle of generation as exhibited between the five elements. Therapy may be applied according to the principles of the "mother-child" law. For example, correcting an energy imbalance within the bladder/kidney unit (water) may be achieved by treating the lungs/large intestine unit (metal); for metal is the "mother" of water. The liver/gallbladder unit (wood) must also be treated, for wood is the "child" of water (kidneys/bladder) and it will absorb the mother's energy if its own energy is not augmented. When treating the lungs/large intestine and liver/gallbladder units, either member of the unit may be treated.

Stimulating the energy flow within the first member of the basic units must also simultaneously coincide with dispersing the energy within the organ or bowel that opposes the organ or bowel receiving the stimulus. Stimulating the energy within the Yin organ of the lungs (metal) must coincide with dispersing the energy within the Yang bowel of the small intestine (fire). According to the law of the five elements, fire destroys metal, or, the small intestine adversely affects the lungs; to neutralize this adverse reaction, the energy within the small intestine (fire) must be dispersed. As a rule, the energy within an organ or bowel that adversely affects another organ or bowel will be found to be naturally superfluous. However if the energy within the small intestine (fire) is not simultaneously neutralized while treating the lungs, that energy will adversely affect the lungs (fire destroys metal) and disrupt the balance between the lungs and large intestine. Consequently the imbalance between the lungs and the large intestine will prevent their conjoint functioning to support the succeeding unit comprised of the bladder/kidneys. Therefore stimulating the energy within either organ or bowel of the basic units must always coincide with neutralizing the energy within any organ or bowel that is in opposition to the basic unit receiving the stimulus. The preceding stimulation-dispersal method must be applied to the following organs and bowel:

Stimulate		*Disperse*
bladder (water)	—	spleen-pancreas (earth)
kidneys (water)	—	stomach (earth)
lungs (metal)	—	small intestine (fire)
large intestine (metal)	—	heart (fire)

(exceptions: heart constrictor, triple heater, liver, gallbladder)

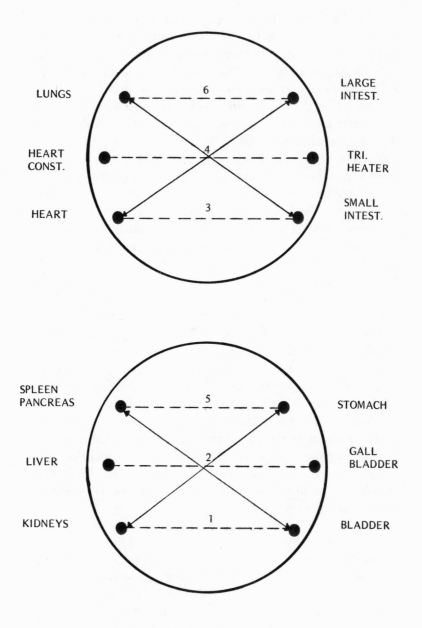

Figure 29. *The Cycles of Generation (Support) and Destruction.*

62

Each of the basic units is the product of the conjoining of a complementary Yin organ and a Yang bowel, i.e. lungs/large intestine. The cycles of interaction between the basic units reflect the two basic cycles of interaction between the earthly elements as they were applied to the individual organs and bowels at the beginning of this section.

THE CYCLE OF DESTRUCTION

adversely affects

1) heart/small intestine (fire)/heart constrictor/ triple heater — lungs/large intestine (metal)

2) lungs/large intestine (metal) — gallbladder/liver (wood)

3) gallbladder/liver (wood) — stomach/spleen-pancreas (earth)

4) stomach/spleen-pancreas (earth) — bladder/kidneys (water)

5) bladder/kidneys (water) — heart/small intestine (fire) heart constrictor/ triple heater

An energy imbalance within an organ or bowel of any of the basic units will result in its adversely affecting, or being adversely affected by, another one of the basic units as illustrated in the cycle of destruction. For example, stimulating the energy within the lungs (metal) during pneumonia must coincide with dispersing the energy with the unit comprised of the heart/small intestine (fire). The energy within the spleen-pancreas/ stomach (earth) must be augmented to enable that unit to support and strengthen the lungs/large intestine metal, cycle of generation). Finally the energy within the bladder/ kidneys must be augmented in order that their being supported by the indisposed lungs/large intestine will not be necessary.

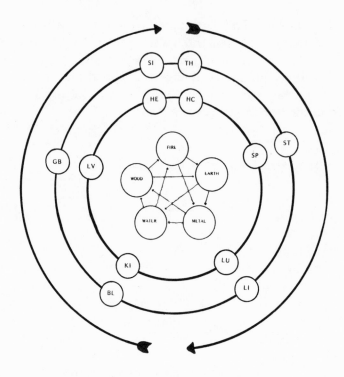

FIGURE 30. *The General Concept of Organs/Bowels and the Five Elements.*

BIORHYTHM

Biorhythm—often referred to as the biological clock—is the regulation of the flow of energy within the body in relation to both solar and lunar time measurement. The word "biorhythm" encompasses all those concepts that denote the natural, inherent pulse underlying all functional aspects of life. In many ways this rhythm is taken for granted because being aware of it would, in a sense, be the same as being constantly aware of the rhythmical basis of one's own breathing. Because it has such a subtle and elusive nature, biorhythm can best be illustrated by exemplifying it when disrupted.

Jet-fatigue—the consequence of suddenly traveling from one time zone to another—is a perfect example of how the body's natural rhythm is disrupted as a result of long-distance travel in a short period of time. It is sometimes difficult to conceive of the body functioning on a strict time schedule until one is abruptly placed in an environment regulated by a *different* schedule. The stress of having to readjust to an environment in relation to time makes one intensely aware of how rigidly scheduled *are* the bodily functions.

Chinese medicine, after observing the circulation of energy throughout the body, formulated biorhythm cycles that precisely account for the energy flow along the meridian circuit during every second of the day. It was discovered that each of the main meridians has two-hour periods during which energy has a maximum and minimum intensity of circulation. For example, between 9 and 11 A.M. energy is at its peak in the spleen-pancreas meridian. Between 11 A.M. and 1 P.M. when the energy activates the heart meridian, it is simultaneously at a minimum intensity in the spleen-pancreas meridian. The following table lists the hours during which energy reaches its peak in each of the organs and bowels and their respective meridians.

TABLE 7. *Biorhythm Cycles.*

1–3 A.M.	Liver
3–5 A.M.	Lung
5–7 A.M.	Large Intestine
7–9 A.M.	Stomach
9–11 A.M.	Spleen-Pancreas
11–1 P.M.	Heart
1–3 P.M.	Small Intestine
3–5 P.M.	Bladder
5–7 P.M.	Kidney
7–9 P.M.	Heart Constrictor
9–11 P.M.	Triple Heater
11–1 A.M.	Gallbladder

Chinese medicine distinguishes little—or not at all—between the ideas of biorhythm, the life-rhythm, and the rhythmical flow of energy throughout the body. Each of these terms implies the idea of a basic, underlying pulsation setting a tempo upon which the myriad functional aspects of life are scheduled. The flow of energy throughout the organs and bowels in accordance with the biorhythm time schedule is essential for a vibrant existence—life itself is a direct indication of unimpeded, rhythmical flow of energy.

Utilizing the biorhythm table will prove to be especially beneficial in the treatment of disease, for it accurately indicates the time during which meridian activity in relation to the organs and bowels is the greatest. For example, a liver malady characterized by paroxysms of pain will respond favorably to various modes of therapy such as needles, acupressure, massage, etc., between the hours of 1:00–3:00 A.M. Asthma attacks will respond to treatment between the hours of 3:00–5:00 A.M. since these are the hours of maximum activity in the lung meridian. Two rules for the application of therapy are:

1) The best time to treat an *excess of energy* is *at*, or *shortly before*, the time of greatest meridian activity.

2) The best time to treat an *energy depletion* is *following* the peak of meridian activity.

5

THE RELATIVISM OF PATHOLOGY

YIN AND YANG

The *Nei Ching* states that "The entire universe is an oscillation of the forces Yin and Yang." While many people who have given much time to the study of Eastern philosophies totally accept this statement as fact, very few have subjectively experienced or understand the elements by which it can be proved valid.

To explain Yin and Yang as they apply to the universe, it is necessary to imagine that state of pure being that preceded the creation of the cosmos. The ancient, sacred manuscripts that talk about the creation of the material universe begin with the question, "What thought could be the only thought that could possibly arise in that infinite state of omnipresence that preceded the creation of the cosmos?" We know that a thought is the result of perceiving an object in the world, but what would be the nature of a thought if the world of objects had not yet been created? The only thought that could possibly arise in that initial state of being would have to be one of self-awareness— there would be no other object in the world for that being to focus its attention on other than on itself. In other words, that initial state of omnipresence became aware of itself as being omnipresent. The first thought then was the exclamation, "I am omnipresent!" It's the same thing that happens when we reflect upon ourselves in a mirror and suddenly become aware of a particular physical characteristic that had been present all the while but which we had taken for granted only because our gaze was always directed outward. A logical second thought was, "Since I am omnipresent, I am all-powerful and can give birth (create) to anything I imagine!" As each thought "died" and another thought was "born," the high intensity energy of each of those thoughts began to vibrate less and less until solid matter, which any scientist will tell you is really energy, resulted. Thus the material world was created by the "birth and death" of thought that "molded" the energy from the initial, infinite source. Many wise men in history, after a sudden flash of illumination have exclaimed, "Why! The whole universe is nothing but a mass of thoughts!" *Yang* is the causative, active, creative principle—life; *Yin* is the resultant, passive, destructive principle—death. The universe is an oscillation of the forces commonly referred to as Yin and Yang.

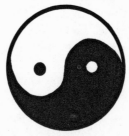

FIGURE 31. *The Symbol of Yin-Yang.*

The relationship of Yin and Yang to that of the whole is often illustrated in another way by equating them to the negative and positive poles within a galvanic current flow; each is separate and distinct in expression, but both are an integral part of the same current. The current could not possibly exist without the bipolarity of its Yin and Yang elements and hence Yin and Yang are distinct and individual but they are also inseparable. Within every object in the universe is the constant, dynamic interaction of these two polar opposites.

The Chinese have extrapolated from the principles regarding the nature of Yin and Yang to consider the feminine as Yin and the masculine as Yang.

> God, Life, Goodness, Justice, Righteousness, Light, Peace, Sun, Heat, Wealth, Happiness, Heaven, High, Raise ... , the active, that which is on the surface, is Yang.
> Devil, Death, Evil, Injustice, Unrighteousness, Darkness, War, Moon, Coldness, Poverty, Unhappiness, Earth, Low, Sink ... , the passive, that which is deep or hidden, is Yin.

Just as we cannot know what heat is if we've never been cold, or what happiness is if we've never been sad, so too Yin and Yang can never exist in total isolation from one another—each is a different side of the same coin; both are constantly interacting and changing. This inseparable dualism persists through all things: foods, attitudes, personal characteristics, thoughts, etc.

Yin and Yang represent every conceivable pair of opposites: birth and death, growth and decay, health and illness, etc. Everything that is born must die, and everything that grows will one day decay, and we can assume that what is Yin today is destined to become Yang in the future, and vice-versa. The relativity of Yin and Yang and the dynamic tension of their interaction are the basis of thought and expression in Chinese philosophy. Maintaining a balance between Yin and Yang results in perfect health of body, mind, and soul.

In terms of medicine, the interaction of Yin and Yang is the basis of the energy pervading and activating the body, and an imbalance in the relativity of Yin and Yang energy is seen as the root of all pathology.

Normal

Imbalance — Less Yin

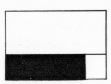
Imbalance — Less Yang

FIGURE 32.

Anatomical Positions of the Body:

Left side is Yang, right side is Yin
Front half is Yin, back half is Yang
Upper half is Yang, lower half is Yin
The surface of the body is Yang, the interior of the body is Yin.

The Six Bowels and the Six Outside Meridians (Bowels' Meridians) are Yang; the Five Organs and Six Inside Meridians (Organs' Meridians and Heart Constrictor Meridian) are Yin.

The body's energy is Yang, the blood is Yin.

As stated earlier, Yin and Yang cannot exist in isolation from one another; neither state as represented by either Yin or Yang is absolute. Therefore, although a bowel such as the stomach or large intestine is said to be Yang, the interior surface of the bowel is Yin. In that every object in the universe exists in relation to its opposite, the relativity of Yin and Yang even applies to the most minute structure of the body—the cell: the cell membrane is Yang, and the cytoplasm is Yin; the nuclear envelope is Yang, the nucleus is Yin.

The Empirical Yin-Yang Concept

In Chinese medicine, Yin is considered to be cold, wet, degenerated, decrepit, ... etc.; Yang is feverish, dry, congested, irritated, inflamed, ... etc. According to Chinese medicine, every disease develops in stages which are characterized by the individual aspects of Yin and Yang. The beginning of a disease is said to be Yang, meaning that it is caloric or progressive, the symptoms are external in the sense that one cannot help but be aware of them. In time, as the disease progresses, the symptoms begin to diminish and the disease usually confines itself to an internal organ, tissue, or nerve; this is the Yin phase. A kidney disease characterized by inflammation of the kidney's surface would be referred to as a kidney/Yang disease; inflammation

TABLE 8. *Yin-Yang Relationships between Tsang-Fu, Inside-Outside and the Meridians.*

		Arm Sunlight Yang	Arm Lesser Yang	Arm Greater Yang	Leg Sunlight Yang	Leg Lesser Yang	Leg Greater Yang
Outside meridian	Meridian	Arm Sunlight Yang	Arm Lesser Yang	Arm Greater Yang	Leg Sunlight Yang	Leg Lesser Yang	Leg Greater Yang
Yang	Bowel	Large Intestine	Triple Heater	Small Intestine	Stomach	Gallbladder	Bladder
Inside meridian	Meridian	Arm Greater Yin	Arm Absolute Yin	Arm Lesser Yin	Leg Greater Yin	Leg Absolute Yin	Leg Lesser Yin
Yin	Organ	Lungs	Heart Constrictor	Heart	Spleen	Liver	Kidney

within the kidney would be referred to as a kidney/Yin disease.

The progression of disease from beginning to end is in six stages:

1) Greater Yang ailment
2) Lesser Yang ailment
3) Sunlight Yang ailment—halfway between Yang and Yin
4) Greater Yin ailment
5) Lesser Yin ailment
6) Absolute Yin ailment—death

Each of these stages lasts anywhere from three to five days, but the stage to which a disease has progressed is often difficult to determine with accuracy because many diseases do not follow the pattern and can go from stage one to stage five without passing through the intermediate stages or passing through too fast to notice. The ability to recognize the aspects of a disease as pertaining to either Yin or Yang will enable a practitioner to administer the correct treatment to bring about a balance of energy within the body.

HSU AND HSIH

In that the universe is an oscillation of the forces Yin and Yang, it is possible to define and classify all life forms, including their individual degrees of functional existence, in terms of one of these two polar opposites. Indeed, the diagnosis of bodily dysfunctions in terms of Yin-Yang energy balance so as to enable us to plot the most promising course of treatment necessitates a thorough understanding of all aspects of this all-inclusive system of classification. No course of treatment can be expected to yield results if the stage to which a pathological condition has progressed cannot be accurately determined in relation to its Yin-Yang energy balance. Only then can a truly personal program of therapy be planned, molded to meet the personal needs of each individual.

But while one may be able to define and classify any condition of the body down to what we can perceive even in an

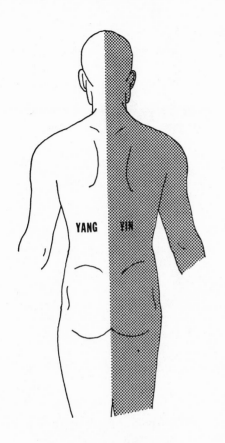

YANG   YIN

FIGURE 33.

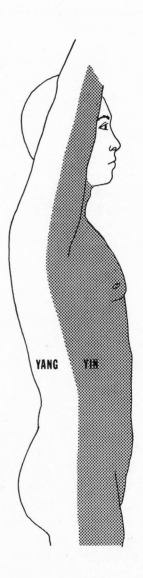

YANG   YIN

FIGURE 34.

73

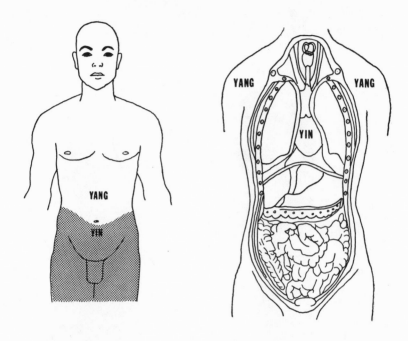

FIGURE 35.   FIGURE 36. *The surface of the body*
is Yang; the inside of the body is Yin.

individual cell in terms of Yin-Yang, that ability will give us
only partial knowledge upon which to formulate a course of
therapy that will have a better-than-average degree of effectiveness. To thoroughly dissect a body, classifying all that we
can see of even its most minute structures within each individual cell will give us knowledge based only on our awareness
of its external aspects—that which we can see with the physical
eye. After peering for hours through an electron microscope in
an effort to find some clue to the cause of a bodily dysfunction,
can it be implied that we could possibly have bypassed
anything? Unfortunately, the answer is "yes." Just as a man may
search for hours for his glasses that all the while have been on
his own nose, so too some men may observe and probe into all
conditions and aspects of the body in searching for the cause of
a disease and may still miss the obvious. We may in all

justification think that we have seen all that can possibly be seen, but have we *seen* that which cannot be seen? To resolve this dilemma, Chinese medicine introduced the concept of Hsu and Hsih.

Hsu and Hsih, like Yin and Yang, represent extremes or opposites. But while Yin and Yang pertain to all that can be perceived or felt by our senses—both physical and mental—Hsu and Hsih pertain to that which, for the most part, can be said to be *invisible*. Therefore Hsu and Hsih take us into a realm much more subtle than that of Yin and Yang in that Hsu and Hsih represent the "energy within the energy" of any object or function. In other words, Hsu and Hsih represent the *intensity* of the energy within any form.

Everything that exists, whether its nature is physiological, anatomical, or inert, is actually a form of energy in that its basic foundation is supported by energy.

The term *Hsu* represents *low-intensity* energy, while *Hsih* represents *high-intensity* energy; energy itself is Yang. The energy that gives one a deathly shock is termed Yang/Hsih; the energy used to give a pleasant massage is Yang/Hsu. With the explanation of Hsu and Hsih we gain knowledge of the most vital factor in the control of bodily functions.

Yin and Yang *indicate* and *generalize*; they are used in relation to external aspects. External is all that can be perceived by both our physical and mental senses, including energy itself. Hsu and Hsih *specify*; they are used in relation to the intensity of the energy that enlivens the external aspects.

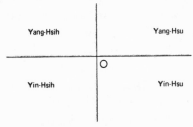

FIGURE 37. *Yin and Yang, and Hsu and Hsih as They Are Applied to Bodily Dysfunctions.*

Constipation is a Yang disease in that it is a result of a bowel—the large intestine. There are two types of constipation: if a person is very strong, having an abundance of high-intensity energy, all the moisture is absorbed from the stool and it is therefore unable to pass from the body; this type of constipation would be termed Yang/Hsih—energy will have to be dispersed. The second type of constipation is one in which the person is very weak and simply has no energy with which to pass the stool; this type is termed Yang/Hsu—energy will have to be augmented.

Diabetes is a Yin disease in that it is the result of an organ—the pancreas. One person eats an over-abundance of rich foods which, as they are digested, create an over-abundance of heat (energy) that taxes, or over-works, the pancreas; this type of Diabetes is termed Yin/Hsih. Another person has a pancreas that cannot perform its function of aiding in digestion; this is a Yin/Hsu form of Diabetes. Many people ask, "If the person with the weak pancreas eats less food, won't the pancreas become stronger as a consequence of not having to work so hard?" This was a therapy used many years ago in treating some diabetics, but as we shall see in the next example, Hsu follows Hsih. Once a chronic Hsu condition develops, it is impossible to regain energy without outside help.

The first step of the common cold is one in which cold, fever, and nasal congestion rack the body. The symptoms are external and all are a form of abnormal high-intensity energy; therefore, the first stage of the common cold is termed Yang/Hsih. In a few days, the symptoms usually internalize and confine themselves mainly to the lungs causing one to cough constantly and to expel phlegm; this stage of the common cold is termed Yin/Hsih. If, in a few more days, the energy of the lungs is depleted in coping with the symptoms, and pneumonia develops, the disease becomes Yin/Hsu. Thus, a disease progresses through stages, each of which is characterized by Hsih followed by Hsu. If the sixth stage which is absolute (Yin/Hsu) develops, the result is death.

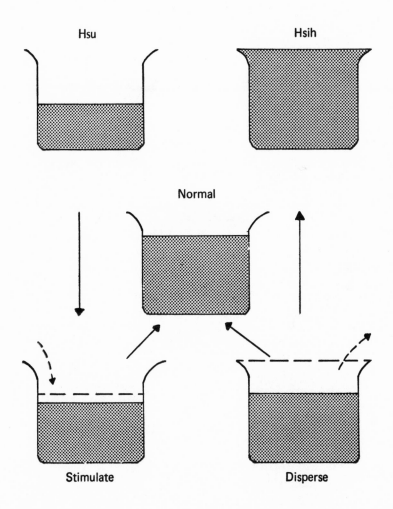

FIGURE 38. *The Relationship Between Yin and Yang, and Hsu and Hsih:* The flow of energy along the meridians should be maintained at a constant level. If the level is excessive it indicates a Hsih condition and energy will have to be dispersed. If the level of energy has been dissipated, a Hsu condition will develop and energy will have to be augmented.

6

ETIOLOGICAL PATHOLOGY

Illness, according to Chinese medicine, indicates an imbalance of energy within the body—the result of a disrupted flow of energy. The conditions which contribute to the disruption of the energy are divided into two categories: internal and external.

1. Internal factors: illness can be caused by excessive emotion and acts.

I A. Excessive anger	II A. Excessive eating
B. Excessive excitement	B. Excessive drinking
C. Excessive thinking	C. Excessive sexual activity
D. Excessive sorrow and anxiety	D. Excessive working
E. Excessive fear	
F. Excessive mourning	
G. Excessive fright (shock)	

2. External factors: illness can be caused by the following natural conditions.

       A. Wind
       B. Cold
       C. Heat
       D. Dampness
       E. Dryness

Excessive wind will affect the liver and nervous systems
Excessive cold will hurt the kidneys and internal gland system
Excessive heat will hurt the spleen-pancreas, bladder, and the
  digestive and lymphatic systems
Excessive dryness will hurt the lungs, skin, and respiratory
system.

Chinese medicine exhibits no great concern about patho-
genic bacteria, for the Chinese believe that it is impossible to
combat the millions of different types of germs in existence. In
accordance with the principles of *preventive medicine*, the
Chinese advocate that the energy within the body be maintained at a *constant level* thereby insuring the body an abundance of natural power to effectively combat any invading
bacteria. Germs can only attack those parts of the body that
have been weakened by any of the preceding internal or
external factors. The Chinese practitioner pays a great deal of
attention to symptoms simply because they reflect a basic
energy imbalance within the body. With proper treatment—as
the energy is balanced—the symptoms will disappear. Viewed
in this way, Chinese medicine may be called *symptomatic*,
meaning that it only uses the symptoms as a gauge to measure
the effectiveness of therapy.

In the West, symptoms are observed, recorded, and analysed;
a name of a disease is attached to the symptoms and therapy—
usually aimed at merely alleviating the symptoms only—
commences. Western medicine then, in the broadest sense of
the word, can be called *terminological*. Unfortunately, though,
if the disease is one that is believed to be *incurable* or *terminal*,
half the battle is already lost because hope, on the part of both
the doctor and the patient, gives way to feelings of futility—or
"what's the use!" By not placing so great an emphasis on the
name of a disease with its inherent negative psychological
implications, but instead eliminating the cause by balancing
the energy, the overall health of the patient will gradually
improve and the symptoms will automatically be eliminated.

7

DIAGNOSIS

Diagnosis is the analysis of symptoms of disease in an effort to determine the basic cause of a disease. With Chinese medicine, along with determining in which organ or bowel a disease is situated, the flow of energy along the main meridians is evaluated; the level of energy within the body, being defined in terms of Hsu and Hsih, is of primary importance in eventually plotting the most effective course of therapy. There are several methods of diagnosis, each reinforcing another; they are: observation, hearing, interrogation, reading the pulse, palpitation of abdominal points, and palpitation of points on the bladder meridian.

OBSERVATION

Observation consists of recognizing all aspects of a patient's external appearance. An experienced practitioner of Chinese medicine will very easily note many clues to the basic cause of a patient's distress in the initial encounter with the patient. An expert practitioner can even draft a general course of therapy by acutely observing the intricate details of facial expression.

Important factors in observation:

1) Color of the face and other parts of the body
2) Indications of an imbalance in diet

3) Condition of the bones, eyes, hair, finger and toe nails, skin and mucosa
4) Coating of tongue and oral fetor
5) Color of urine, stool, and other secretions

In general, the color of the face and other parts of the body is indicative of a specific organ or bowel and its physiological function, and also the degree of meridian involvement. For example, a blackish tone on the inside of the forearm and around the eyebrows indicates a kidney and/or an internal gland dysfunction. Chinese medicine lists five colors as representative of the organs and bowels, and their functions; they are:

1) Black—kidneys, bladder, and internal glands; especially a sexual hormone imbalance;
2) Red—heart, brain, and blood vessels;
3) White—lungs, skin, and respiratory system;
4) Yellow—spleen-pancreas, stomach, and lymphatic system;
5) Green—liver, and nervous system.

HEARING

The Chinese method of diagnosis by hearing should not be confused with the Western method in which mechanical devices are used. Chinese practitioners use no mechanical devices, but are advised to maintain a "proper" distance (3–4 feet) from the patient. A constant effort to go beyond merely listening to the patient must be exerted. Important factors in hearing:

1) The general volume of the voice and the force behind it
   a) loud and strong
   b) low and weak
2) Aspects of breathing
   a) coughing and panting
3) Water and/or gas sounds in the stomach and intestines

As in observation, the voice of the patient can also be linked to a specific organ depending upon its quality.

1) Shouting, or calling-out quality—liver
2) Laughing quality—heart
3) Singing quality—spleen-pancreas
4) Crying quality—lungs
5) Sighing quality—kidneys

INTERROGATION

This method of diagnosis is very similar to the Western method. Important factors in interrogation:

1) Patient's complaints
2) Previous medical history
3) Family medical history
4) Symptoms
5) Syndrome
6) Appetite
7) Excretion

Chinese medicine takes all feelings into consideration whether they are physical or emotional in that they are vital clues enabling the practitioner to develop an understanding of the different needs of each individual. Feelings that are especially significant are: heat and coldness, pain and soreness, dizziness, sensations on the tips of the fingers and toes, feelings experienced in various dreams, and depth of sleep. Some purely physical factors are: sweat, menstrual cycle, thirst, emesis, epistaxis, and bleeding.

READING THE PULSES

The method of reading the pulses as developed in Chinese medicine is one of the greatest contributions to diagnostic procedures. No other method of diagnosis has such all-encompassing scope in indicating the overall state of energy balance within the body. The ultra-sensitivity of this method enables a practitioner to diagnose the subtlest fluctuations in the flow of energy between the organs and bowels along the meridian circuit. The development of a superior ability to read the pulses demands a complete understanding of the basic techniques and, even more important, the seizing of every opportunity that arises to apply those techniques. In reading the pulses, scholarship, thorough though it may be, is no substitute for actual experience.

Each one of the organs and bowels, the main meridians, and the heart constrictor is reflected at the radial artery and can be felt as a pulse at the wrist. (The meridians Jen-Mo and Tu-Mo are exceptions, for they exist outside the general energy circulatory system.) To determine the exact position of the pulses, first locate the middle (or kuan) pulse which is at the level of the styloid protuberance and place the third finger atop it; second, locate the top (or tsun) pulse which lies between the fold of the wrist and the styloid protuberance; third, locate the bottom (or ch'ih) pulse beneath the kuan. The distance between the middle and the top pulse is equal to the distance between the middle and the bottom pulse.

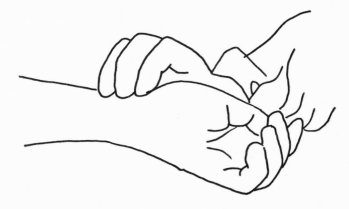

FIGURE 39.

Following are the locations of the pulses on the wrists, and the organs and bowels they reflect:

LEFT WRIST (YANG)		RIGHT WRIST (YIN)	
Superficial	*Deep*	*Deep*	*Superficial*
small intestine	heart	lungs	large intestine
gallbladder	liver	spleen-pancreas	stomach
bladder	kidneys	heart constrictor	triple heater

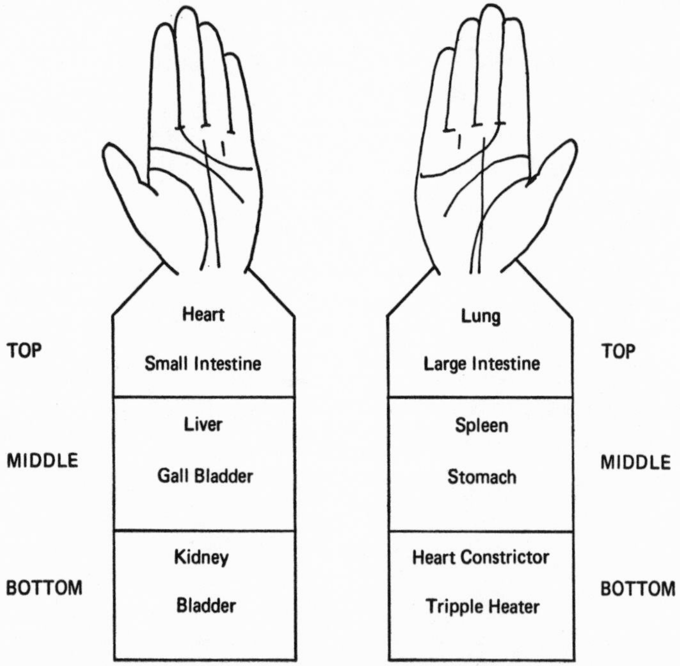

TOP	Heart	Lung	TOP	
	Small Intestine	Large Intestine		
MIDDLE	Liver	Spleen	MIDDLE	
	Gall Bladder	Stomach		
BOTTOM	Kidney	Heart Constrictor	BOTTOM	
	Bladder	Tripple Heater		

FIGURE 40.

There are 27 pulse indications as expounded in *Chang Chung-Ching* B.C. 180), but eight will usually suffice for the ordinary diagnosis. The eight indications are: fast, slow, vast, weak, slippery, astringent, tight but thin, tardy—irregular—often skipping a beat.

Quality	Diagnosis	Therapy
FAST—more than six beats to each respiration	fever	disperse
SLOW—five or fewer beats	cold, acute pain, general fatigue	stimulate
VAST—swollen, strong, full	excess in Heart Constr. or and Triple Heater	disperse
WEAK—soft, deep	malnutrition, palsy, decrease of energy	stimulate
SLIPPERY—floating, superficial	fever, superficial complaints	stimulate
ASTRINGENT—deep, strong	excess Yin	disperse
TIGHT BUT THIN—stretched	liver and bile ailments, epigastric pain, headaches, satiated	disperse
TARDY—IRREGULAR—OFTEN SKIPPING A BEAT	excess of Yang and lack of Yin	stimulate Yin

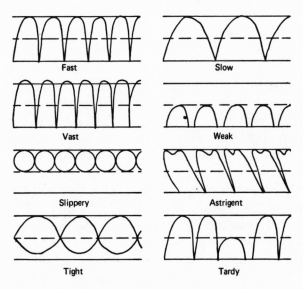

FIGURE 41. *The Eight Ordinary Pulses.*

At each location two pulses are indicated: the superficial, or surface pulse, corresponds to the Yang bowels; the sunken, or deep pulse, corresponds to the Yin organs and heart constrictor.

The pulses will also indicate an impeded energy flow along any of the 12 main meridians in that a dysfunction of an organ or bowel correlates to the energy flow along its respective meridian. Light pressure is used to detect the surface pulses; strong pressure is used to detect the deep pulses.

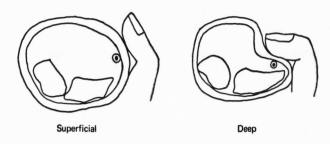

Superficial   Deep

FIGURE 42.

A practitioner who after years of experience develops an expertise in reading the pulse deserves the utmost respect. A proficiency in pulse reading not only enables the practitioner to determine the most minute energy imbalance within the body at the time of the diagnosis, but also supplies him with knowledge of disease suffered in the past. *He can therefore predict pathological conditions which can be expected in the future, for they will be the outcome of the present conditions of the body which are the outcome of the past.*

Reading the pulses is by far the most sensitive diagnostic procedure in the world today. The series of clinical and laboratory tests administered to determine the cause or causes of pathological conditions—along with being very expensive—often yield no tangible results because they lack sensitivity. Often a patient is obviously ill, but it may be impossible to determine the cause of his distress by orthodox medical practices; in such cases reading the pulses is invaluable for it presents the entelechy of disease rather than the disease itself. The symptoms are those of the pre-clinical stage of disease and it may be years before they are seen as an overt disease.

The Pulses of Pregnancy

If the bottom pulse is very strong—almost beating against the finger—and completely different from that of the top and bottom positions, or, if the top pulse (heart) on the left wrist is very fluent, the lady *is* pregnant. If the top pulses, regardless of how deeply they are pressed, are rapid, slippery, and tight, the pregnancy is in the third month. When the top and bottom pulses cease to be slippery but remain rapid no matter how firmly they are pressed, the pregnancy is in the fifth month. If the top and bottom pulses on the left wrist are more rapid than the pulses on the right wrist, the child will be a male; if the pulses are more rapid on the right wrist, the child will be a female.

PALPATION OF ABDOMINAL POINTS

An energy imbalance within an organ or bowel will affect the entire length of its meridian causing it—and especially the individual points on that meridian—to become sensitive to external pressure. Palpation is applied to the points of the meridians on the abdomen to determine an imbalance of energy within any of the viscera and also to confirm or negate a diagnosis that has been made by reading the pulses. Palpation of points on the abdomen is the easiest way to detect an abnormal energy balance and—along with reading the pulses—it is a standard diagnostic procedure of Chinese medicine.

Steps in palpation of abdominal points:

1) The practitioner caressingly passes his palm over the entire surface of the abdomen
2) Variations in the overall temperature should be noted
3) Areas that are unusually hard, soft, and tense or tight should be noted
4) Light finger pressure is used to detect areas that are unusually sensitive and painful

Points: warmer, tight or tense, acute pain—Hsih (excess energy)

cooler, soft and hyposensitive—Hsu (insufficient energy)

Along with indicating the energy balance within the viscera, palpation of points on the meridians will provide a knowledge of the energy balance in relation to the external senses also:

1) Lung meridian—nose, throat, lungs
2) Large intestine meridian—mouth, tongue, nose, face, ears, eyes, throat, esophagus, stomach
3) Heart meridian—heart, central nervous system
4) Small intestine meridian—head, nape of neck, back, elbows
5) Stomach meridian—viscera in general
6) Spleen-pancreas meridian—intestines, stomach, liver, spleen, lungs

PALPATION OF POINTS ON THE BLADDER MERIDIAN

There are 12 points—the *iu* points—on the bladder meridian that correlate to each one of the organs, bowels, and heart constrictor and can therefore be palpated to determine the energy balance within any of the viscera and their respective meridians. Pressure applied to these points will elicit a definite reaction of pain if the energy within the organ identified with that point is imbalanced. The points on the bladder meridian, along with being *diagnostic* points, are also *treatment* points for the specific organ or bowel with which they are identified. The *iu* points are: lungs, B 13; large intestine, B 25; stomach, B 21; spleen-pancreas, B 20; heart, B 15; small intestine, B 27; bladder, B 28; kidneys, B 23; liver, B 18; gallbladder, B 19; triple heater, B 22; heart constrictor, B 14.

8

THE TECHNIQUE OF ACUPUNCTURE

THE POSITION OF THE PATIENT'S BODY

When administering acupuncture treatments, the following three rules must be strictly adhered to:

1) The patient *must* be comfortable
2) The points *must* be clearly visible
3) The patient *must* be in such a position that any adjustments, manipulations, etc., can be easily carried out

FIGURE 43.

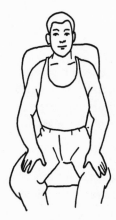

Sitting position 1

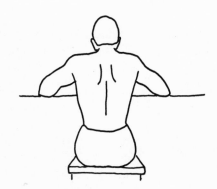

Sitting position 2

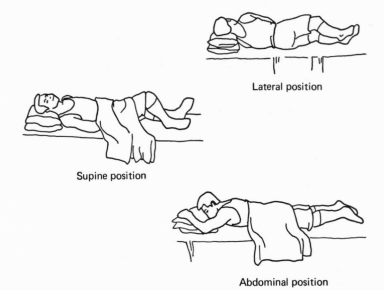

Lateral position

Supine position

Abdominal position

LOCALIZATION OF THE POINTS

Methods of Finger Measurement

In Chinese medicine, the basic unit of measurement is the "tsun," or the Chinese inch. The length of the tsun is relative; it varies from individual to individual and therefore can also be called the "living" inch. The following methods use *the width of the patient's fingers* as standard measure for the location of points:

a. The middle finger measurement
When the patient forms a ring by joining his middle finger to his thumb, the inside distance between the first and second joints of the middle finger is 1 tsun

b. The thumb measurement

The width of the first joint of the thumb is 1 tsun

c. The combined finger measurement
    The width of the second joint of the index and the middle finger is 2 tsun: the preceding, plus the ring finger and the little finger linked together is 3 tsun

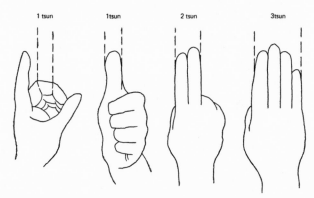

FIGURE 44. *Methods of Finger Measurement*

Methods of Bone-Convertible Measurement

These methods are used for determining the fixed length between the different regions of the body:

a. between the middle of the eyebrows and the middle of the natural line of hair on the forehead is 3 tsun

b. The distance between the middle of the natural line of the hair on the forehead and the middle of the natural line of the hair at the back of the head is 12 tsun

c. The distance between the middle of the natural line of the hair at the back of the head and the seventh cervical vertebra is 3 tsun

d. The distance between the two mastoid processes on the posterior side of the auricle is 9 tsun

e. The distance between the jugular notch and the costophrenic angle is 9 tsun

f. The distance between the middle of the nipples of the breasts is 8 tsun

g. The distance between the xiphoid process and the umbilicus is 8 tsun
h. The distance between the umbilicus and the superior border of the symphysis pubis is 5 tsun
i. The distance between the anterior axillary fold and the elbow crease is 12 tsun
j. The distance between the elbow crease and the wrist crease is 12 tsun
k. The distance between the greater trochanter of the femur and the later patella is 19 tsun
l. The distance between the middle of the popliteal fossa and the superior border of the lateral malleolus is 16 tsun
m. The distance between the superior border of the lateral malleolus and inferior border of the heel is 3 tsun

NEEDLING

Before any treatment, a practitioner should thoroughly inspect all needles to determine that they are in perfect condition. All needles should be straight and fine and special attention should be given to the joint at which the body of the needle meets the root (chapter 1, figure 2); all abnormal needles should be discarded. Needles should always be sterilized prior to treatment with alcohol or steam.

If, during the course of the treatment, a patient becomes pale, suddenly unconscious, or begins to perspire profusely, all needles should be withdrawn immediately and the patient should be made to lie at an angle with his head lower than his feet. A mild condition can be remedied by giving the patient a drink of water; a serious one—such as sudden unconsciousness—can be remedied by inserting a needle into any one of the points: Jenchung (TU 26), Nei Kuan (P 6), Chungchung (P 9), Tsu-san-li (S 36); stimulating any one of these points will restore consciousness.

The Method of Stimulation

1) Massage the point to be treated prior to inserting the needle
2) Insert the needle slowly in stages
3) Pique the points on the meridian in the direction of the flow of energy along the meridian
4) Keep the needle in place for three to twenty minutes and then slowly withdraw it in stages

The Method of Dispersal

1) *Do not massage* the point to be treated
2) Insert the needle deeply and withdraw it rapidly using a strong, twisting motion
3) Pique the points on the meridian in the opposite direction of the flow of energy along the meridian
4) Keep the needle in place for only a few seconds

Angles of Insertion of Needles

1) Vertical insertion(90°)—suitable for regions of abundant musculature
2) Slanting insertion(30°–60°)—suitable for areas on the chest and back
3) Transversal insertion(10°–20°)—suitable for head and superficial regions

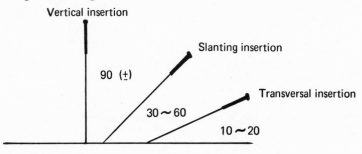

FIGURE 45. *Diagram of the angles of needle insertion.*

Teh-chi

After a needle has been inserted, the patient may report a distinct sensation at the point being piqued which often is difficult to describe accurately. In Chinese medicine this sensation is called Teh-chi and it is considered essential in that it is an indication that the treatment will be effective.

On the part of the patient, Teh-chi denotes those distinct subjective feelings that arise at the point being punctured. There are a variety of sensations but usually soreness, heaviness, tightness, and expansion predominate. To the acupuncturist, Teh-chi denotes actual sensations of resistance and palpable motion of the impaling needle—a sensation as though the needle is being "sucked" into the tissue.

Every two or three minutes the needle should be half-rotated in a counterclockwise direction by using the thumb and index finger to grasp the needle head. This will in no way injure the tissue of the body. Often a patient will report a sensation of diffusion and conduction around the point as the needle is rotated; this is a secondary effect of stimulation.

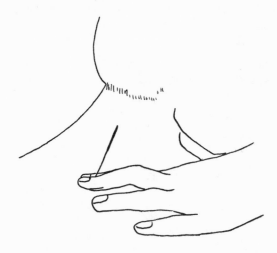

FIGURE 46

CONDITIONS PROHIBITING THE USE OF NEEDLES

The following diseases and special cases are excluded from needling treatment: patients who suffer from serious hemorrhagic diseases, local malignant tumor, over-exertion, an overfull or empty stomach, acute exhaustion, cardiac conditions, and extremely sensitive constitutions. Hoku (LI 4), Tsu-san-li (S 36), Yin-chio (SP 6), and all points over the abdomen should be avoided during pregnancy.

ACUPRESSING AND MERIDIAN MASSAGE

Smoothing or Pushing	○ Rubbing or Palm Pressing
Picking	● Finger Pressing or Thumb Pressing

FIGURE 47. *Signs of Acupressing*

Pressing. Always press firmly with a forward, downward motion using the bulb of the thumb or the palm of the hand. The elbow is used for intense pain in the muscles and joints since the pressure is stronger and penetrates more deeply.

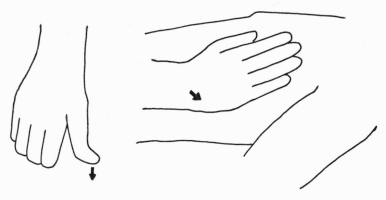

FIGURE 48.

Soothing Stimulation. Using the bulb of the thumb, the fingers, or the palm of the hand, massage with a light and rapid motion. The end result of this type of massage on painful areas of the body can be described as a soothing stimulation.

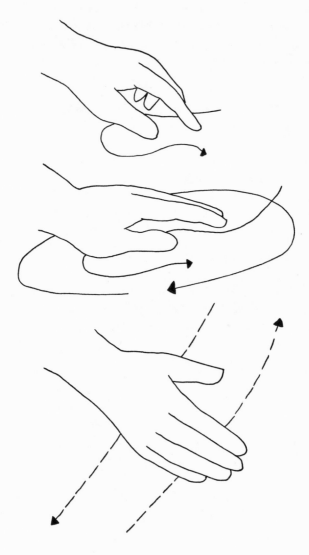

FIGURE 49.

Pushing. Only use the bulb of the thumb to stimulate or disperse the meridians on the back and the extremities—the arms and the back. Usually pushing is applied in series of 100-300 strokes at one treatment session; baby oil or ginger juice can be used for lubrication.

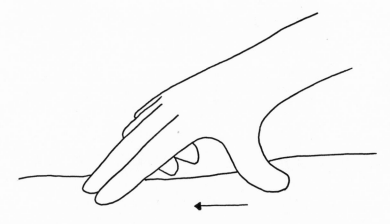

FIGURE 50.

Picking. Use the thumb and index finger to pick up the skin along with the muscle on areas such as the neck, upper back, face, and along the spinal column.

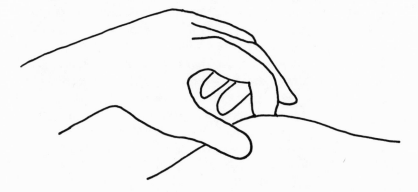

FIGURE 51.

Rubbing. Use the thumbs, fingers *and* palms. Both hands can be used simultaneously to rub the arms and legs. This method is very effective for arthritis.

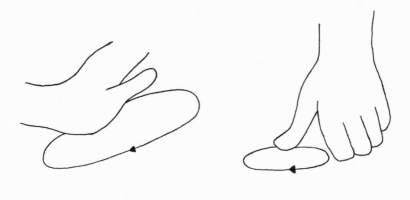

FIGURE 52.   FIGURE 53.

There is a traditional Chinese habit of turning walnuts around in the hands to promote the circulation of blood in the arms, hands, and all the way to the tips of the fingers. Because blood flows to the area of the body in active use at the moment, when one thinks, it flows to the brain; when one walks, it flows to the feet. The Chinese believe that the use of the hands tends to promote a feeling of mental serenity, for the blood flowing to the hands lessens the strain on the brain and consequently one is less prone to states of overemotionalism. For example, in self-treatment for insomnia—which is usually the clatter of one's own thoughts keeping one awake—lie with the feet stretched out and point the toes downward and then upward as far as possible to stimulate the flow of blood in the lower limbs. Finally, rub the palms of the hands together and massage the area around the navel 100-300 times. Sound sleep is assured.

THE POINTS OF THE EAR

The delicate beauty inherent in the structure of the human ear likens this organ of the body to a work of art beside which any other masterpiece would stand second. Few people realize that the surface of the ear contains points for every single part of the entire human body. Because of its intricacy, the ear is the least understood of all the organs of the body.

Although the points of the ear as they correlate to the various parts of the body have been accurately determined, the final results of acupuncture when applied to the ear points vary. Often the needling of two or more points will have an entirely different effect than that logically anticipated. Part II lists the individual ear points and Part III contains time-tested prescriptions for specific ailments using a combination of ear points. But ear points should never entirely take the place of body points when treating any disease.

Palpation of the ear points with an object such as the tapered top of a pen will accurately indicate a disturbance in the energy balance of the organ or bowel that is identified with the point. For this reason, palpation of the ear points is widely used as a diagnostic procedure to reinforce other methods of diagnosis.

The terms "stimulation" and "dispersal" do not apply to the points on the ear as they do to the points on the body. With the ear, needles are inserted and the effects are observed and noted before the next step of therapy is planned. Since there are few standard rules regarding a definite course of therapy to follow, knowledge, wisdom, and experience on the part of the therapist must necessarily dictate one's actions when treating the ear.

The ear can truly be called the wilderness of the body for the ear points are relatively new to us and it is therefore necessary to await the results of present-day research before theories can be developed and therapies standarized. The results obtained thus far do however suggest that a vast new world of knowledge is contained within the apparent fragile structure of the ear.

PART II

Acupuncture Points

FOREWORD

Part II lists the common acupuncture points that are available for the specific ailments listed under "indications." Several points are "available" meaning that you must choose which point or points you will use, and that choice is dependent upon the various aspects of each person's ailment. The combination of points decided upon for a specific ailment is called a "prescription" and your ability to create an effective prescription will depend upon how thoroughly you have assimilated the basic principles of Part I.

In China, when a prescription was formulated that was unusually effective in the treatment of a disease, it became a closely guarded secret of the physician who created it. This secret prescription was passed on to a son if he decided to follow in his father's footsteps. The physician had so thoroughly studied and understood the basic principles of his healing art that he had developed an intuitive sense of knowing exactly which points to combine—or prescribe —for specific diseases. It was totally different from modern practices which often prescribe penicillin for the same condition in five different people without considering the needs of the individual or the other at present unnoticeable effects of such therapy.

Diagnosis—using all of the various procedures—is the first step in the eventual formulation of a prescription. Having determined in which meridian or meridians there is an energy imbalance, the next step is to decide upon a pattern that will include those meridians to be treated to balance the energy. Finally, after studying the various points on the meridians to be treated, you must choose the specific points to be stimulated and dispersed—at which time the prescription is complete.

The formulation of a prescription is an art; just as an artist has several colors from which to choose, so too, there are often several points from which to choose for treating a single ailment. And just as an artist visualizes his final masterpiece, in the same manner you must anticipate the end result of your treatment. This is not difficult if the cycles of interaction between the organs and bowels as they reflect the interaction between the elements form the basis for your prescription.

Acupuncture enables you to actively contact and manipulate the basic life force—the invisible energy within the body, and *you must constantly strive to see that which cannot be seen*—the energy balance or imbalance within the body. However do not ignore or relegate to secondary importance the apparent symptoms of a disease, for symptoms are crucial in that they are signposts to direct your gaze.

9

ACUPUNCTURE POINTS

THE FIVE ELEMENT POINTS

Each of the twelve main meridians has five element points that are treated according to the "mother-child" law explained in Part I. Energy within a merician can be augmented by treating its "mother" point which correlates to the element that *produces* the element with which the meridian is identified. For instance, augmenting the flow of energy along the spleen-pancreas meridian would be accomplished by treating SP2, for SP2 is the fire point in the spleen-pancreas meridian (earth) and according to the law of the five elements fire produces earth, or, fire is the "mother" of earth. Energy along a meridian is dispersed by treating the "child" point which correlates to the element *succeeding or following* the element with which the meridian is identified. For instance, overactivity along the meridian would be remedied by treating SP5, for SP5 is the metal point on the spleen-pancreas meridian; earth produces metal, or, metal is the "child" of earth.

TABLE 9. *The Five Elements and Transmitting Points.*

	Kuan-chung (TH-1)	Yi-mien (TH-2)	Chung-tu (TH-3)	Chi-kou (TH-6)	Tien-ching (TH-10)
Triple Heater (Yang Minister Fire)	Kuan-chung (TH-1)	Yi-mien (TH-2)	Chung-tu (TH-3)	Chi-kou (TH-6)	Tien-ching (TH-10)
Stomach (Yang Earth)	Li-tui (S-45)	Nei-ting (S-44)	Hsen-ku (S-43)	Chue-hsi (S-41)	Tsu-san-li (S-36)
Small Intestine (Yang Prince Fire)	Shio-tse (SI-1)	Cheng-ku (SI-2)	Hou-hsi (SI-3)	Yang-ku (SI-5)	Shiao-hai (SI-8)
Gallbladder (Yang Wood)	Chiao-ming (GB-44)	Hsia-hsi (GB-43)	Ling-chi (GB-41)	Yang-fu (GB-38)	Yang-ling-chuan (GB-34)
Bladder (Yang Water)	Che-yin (B-67)	Tung-ku (B-66)	Su-ku (B-65)	Kuen-lung (B-60)	Wei-chung (B-40)
Large Intestine (Yang Metal)	Shan-yang (LI-1)	Er-chien (LI-2)	San-chien (LI-3)	Yang-hsi (LI-5)	Chui-chih (LI-11)
Yang Meridians — 5 Elements	Metal	Water	Wood	Fire	Earth
5 Transmitting Points	Source Points	Stream Points	Cataract Points	River Points	Sea Points
Yin Meridians — 5 Elements	Wood	Fire	Earth	Metal	Water
Liver (Yin Wood)	Ta-tueng (LV-1)	Hsin-chien (LV-2)	Tai-chung (LV-3)	Chung-fung (LV-4)	Chui-chuan (LV-8)
Heart (Yin Prince fire)	Shiao-chung (H-9)	Shiao-fu (H-8)	Shen-men (H-7)	Ling-tao (H-4)	Shiao-hai (H-3)
Spleen-Pancreas (Yin Earth)	Yin-pai (SP-1)	Ta-tu (SP-2)	Tai-pai (SP-3)	Shan-chiu (SP-5)	Yin-ling-chuan (SP-9)
Lung (Yin Metal)	Shiao-shan (L-11)	Yui-chi (L-10)	Tai-yuan (L-9)	Ching-chiu (L-8)	Chih-tse (L-5)
Kidney (Yin Water)	Yung-chuan (K-1)	Jan-ku (K-2)	Tai-hsi (K-3)	Fu-liu (K-7)	Yin-ku (K-10)
Heart Constrictor (Yin Minister Fire)	Chung-chung (HC-9)	Lao-kung (HC-8)	Ta-ling (HC-7)	Chien-she (HC-5)	Chui-tse (HC-3)

THE FIVE TRANSMITTING POINTS

The gamut covered from the source points to the sea points correlates exactly to the various degrees of seriousness of a specific disease in reference to the organ or bowel with which any one of the points is identified. The source point is treated for superficial and acute diseases in accordance with the concept that the source from which water flows to the sea is shallow; the sea point is treated for diseases that are very serious, long term, or chronic, for the sea point designates the point at which the flow of water achieves its maximum depth, or power.

POINTS OF ORIGIN AND POINTS ON THE POSTERIOR AND ANTERIOR SIDES OF THE BODY

An energy imbalance within an organ or bowel and its respective meridian can be remedied by treating its point of origin in addition to one of various points on the front or back of the body that is identified with the diseased organ or bowel. Points on the front of the body are utilized when the patient is lying on his back; those on the back, when the patient is lying on his stomach (all of the treatment points for the organs and bowels as listed on the back lie on the Bladder Meridian). Treating the point of origin of a specific organ or bowel reinforces the effects of therapy applied to any of the other points also being treated (front or back) in reference to the same organ or bowel; therefore, when treating a point on the front or back, the point of origin is always included.

THE CONJUNCTIVE POINTS

The conjunctive points lie on the extremities and conjoin the meridians of the basic organ/bowel units. Treating the conjunctive points strengthens the relationship between the meridians of the basic organ/ bowel units which they conjoin.

TABLE 10. *Associating Points.*

Meridians	Organ (bowel) Points		Origin Points	Conjunctive Points	Assembling Points
	Back	Front			
Lung	Fei-shu (B-13)	Chung-fu (L-1)	Tai-yuan (L-9)	Lei-chieh (L-7)	Kung-tsue (L-6)
Large Intestine	Ta-chang-shu (B-25)	Tien-shu (S-25)	Ho-ku (LI-4)	Pien-li (LI-6)	Wung-liu (LI-7)
Stomach	Wei-shu (B-21)	Chung-wan (JEN-12)	Chung-yang (S-42)	Fung-lung (S-40)	Liong-chiu (S-34)
Spleen Pancreas	Pi-shu (B-20)	Chang-men (K-13)	Tai-pai (SP-3)	Ta-pao (SP-21) Kung-sun (SP-4)	Ti-chi (SP-8)
Heart	Hsin-shu (B-15)	Chu-chuei (JEN-14)	Shen-men (H-7)	Tung-li (H-5)	Yin-hsi (H-6)
Small Intestine	Shiao-chang-shu (B-27)	Kuan-yuan (JEN-4)	Wan-ku (SI-4)	Chi-cheng (SI-7)	Yang-lao (SI-6)
Bladder	Pan-kuang-shu (B-28)	Chung-chi (JEN-3)	Ching-ku (B-64)	Fei-yang (B-58)	Jing-men (B-63)
Kidney	Shen-shu (B-23)	Ching-men (GB-25)	Tai-hsi (K-3)	Ta-chung (K-4)	Shui-chuan (K-5)
Heart Constrictor	Chueh-yin-shu (B-14)	Shan-chung (JEN-17)	Ta-ling (HC-7)	Nei-kuan (HC-6)	Hsi-men (HC-4)
Triple Heater	San-chiao-shu (B-22)	She-men (JEN-5)	Yang-chih (TH-4)	Wai-kuan (TH-5)	Hui-chung (TH-7)
Gallbladder	Tan-shu (B-19)	Jih-yueh (GB-24)	Chiu-hsi (GB-40)	Kuang-ming (GB-37)	Wai-chiu (GB-36)
Liver	Kan-shu (B-18)	Chi-men (LV-14)	Tai-chung (LV-3)	Li-kou (LV-5)	Chung-tu (LV-6)

THE ASSEMBLING POINTS

The assembling points are high-energy centers. Treating the assembling points releases an additional supply of energy along the meridians to the organ or bowel with which they are identified.

THE EIGHT SPECIAL MEETING POINTS

The eight special meeting points are utilized to treat serious conditions which exist in relation to a general system of the body. For example, an energy imbalance within one or several organs will respond favorably to treatment applied to individual points on the meridians in which the imbalance has been diagnosed in addition to treating the point Chang-men (LV 13) which is designated as the Organ Meeting Point. LV13 is designated as the Organ Meeting Point because it exerts a special influence over all the bowels of the body.

TABLE 11. *The Eight Special Meeting Points.*

Organ Meeting Point	Chang-men (LV-13)
Bowel Meeting Point	Chung-wan (JEN-12)
Energy Meeting Point	Shang-chung (JEN-17)
Blood Meeting Point	Ke-shu (B-17)
Pulse Meeting Point	Tai-yuan (L-9)
Marrow Meeting Point	Hsuan-chung (GB-39)
Nerve Meeting Point	Yang-ling-chuan (GB-34)
Bone Meeting Point	Ta-shu (B-11)

THE MEETING POINTS OF THE EIGHT
EXTRAORDINARY MERIDIANS

The points at which the eight extraordinary meridians intersect one another can be treated to simultaneously affect the flow of energy to several internal or external organs and bowels.

TABLE 12. *The Meeting Points of the Eight Extraordinary Meridians.*

Kung-sun (SP-4) Nei-Kuan (HC-6)	Chung-mo Yin-wei-mo	flow into stomach, heart and chest.
Hou-hsi (SI-3) Shen-mo (B-62)	Tu-mo Yang-chiao-mo	flow into eyes, ears, head, neck, shoulder, small intestine and bladder.
Tsu-ling-chi (GB-41) Wai-kuan (TH-5)	Tai-mo Yang-wei-mo	flow into eyes, ears, chin, neck and shoulder.
Lee-chueh (L-7) Chiao-hai (K-6)	Jen-mo Yin-chiao-mo	flow into chest, throat, and lungs.

10

ACUPUNCTURE POINTS ON THE ABDOMINAL REGION

See figures

1. TA-HENG (SP 15)

   LOCATION: 3.5 tsun beside the umbilicus along the lateral side of the retus abdominis muscle.

   ANATOMY: MUSCLE: External oblique, internal oblique and transverse of the abdomen.
   NERVE: 10th intercostal.

   MERIDIAN: Belongs to the Leg Greater Yin (spleen) meridian and is the meeting point of the Leg Greater Yin (spleen) meridian and Yang-Wei-Mo.

   INDICATIONS: Abdominal distention, constipation, diarrhea, dysentery, intestinal paralysis, lenkorrhagia, ascariasis.

2. FU-SHE (SP 13)

   LOCATION: Above the inguinal region, 7 fen over Chung-men and 3.5 tsun beside the mid-abdominal line.

   ANATOMY: MUSCLE: Aponcurosis of external oblique, internal oblique and lower part of the transverse muscle of the abdomen.
   NERVE: Femoral nerve arising from L2-L4.

MERIDIAN: Belongs to the Leg Greater Yin (spleen) meridian and is the meeting point of the Leg Greater Yin (spleen), the Leg Absolute Yin (liver) meridians and Yin-Wei-Mo.

INDICATIONS: Appendicitis, constipation, rupture.

3. CHUNG-MEN (SP 12)

LOCATION: On the lateral side of the femoral artery, superior border of the symphysis pubis and 3.5 tsun beside the mid-abdominal line.

ANATOMY: MUSCLE: Aponeurosis of external oblique.
NERVE: Lateral cutaneous of the femoral nerve arising from L1-L4, muscle branch of the femoral and trunk of the femoral nerve.

MERIDIAN: Belongs to the Leg Greater Yin (spleen) meridian and is the meeting point of the Leg Greater Yin (spleen) and the Leg Absolute Yin (liver) meridians.

INDICATIONS: Orchitis, endometritis, rupture, hernia of the cord.

4. CHANG-MEN (LV 13)

LOCATION: Below the end of the 11th rib, where it meets the mid-axillary line.

ANATOMY: MUSCLE: Internal oblique, external oblique, and transverse muscles of the abdomen.
NERVE: 10th intercostal nerve.

MERIDIAN: Belongs to the Leg Absolute Yin (liver) meridian, is the meeting point of the Leg Absolute Yin (liver) and the Leg Lesser Yang (gallbladder) meridians.

INDICATIONS: Hepatitis, peritonitis, ascites, vomiting, emesis.

5. TAI-MO (GB 26)

LOCATION: At the same level with the umbilicus, directly below Chang-men.

ANATOMY: MUSCLE: Internal oblique, external oblique, transverse muscle of abdomen.
NERVE: 12th intercostal nerve.

MERIDIAN: Belongs to the Leg Lesser Yang (gallbladder) meridian and is the meeting point of the Leg Lesser Yang (gallbladder) meridian and Tai-Mo.

INDICATIONS: Cystitis, endametritis, irregular menstruation.

6. WU-SHU (GB 27)

LOCATION: 3 tsun below Tai-Mo about 1 tsun in front of the antero-superior iliac spine.

ANATOMY: MUSCLE: Internal oblique, external oblique, transverse muscle of abdomen.
NERVE: Iliohypogastric nerve arising from L1.

MERIDIAN: Belongs to the Leg Lesser Yang (gallbladder) meridian and is the meeting point of the Leg Lesser Yang (gallbladder) meridian and Tai-Mo.

INDICATIONS: Orchitis, endometritis, lumbago, abdominal pain.

7. WEI-TAO (GB 28)

LOCATION: On the antero-inferior part of the anterior superior iliac spine and ½ tsun right below Wu-Shu.

ANATOMY: MUSCLE: Internal oblique, external oblique, transverse muscles of the abdomen.
NERVE: Ilio inguinal nerve arising from L1.

MERIDIAN: Belongs to the Leg Lesser Yang (gallbladder) meridian and is the meeting point of the Leg Lesser Yang (gallbladder) meridian and Tai-mo.

INDICATIONS: Habitual constipation, endometritis, gripping pain.

8. CHIU-WEI (JEN 15)

LOCATION: On the mid-abdominal line, ½ tsun below the xiphoid process.

ANATOMY: NERVE: 6th intercostal nerve.

MERIDIAN: Lo point of Jen-Mo.

INDICATIONS: Pain in the stomach region, madness, high blood pressure, murmurs, cardiopathia.

9. CHUNG-WEN (JEN 12)

LOCATION: On the mid-abdominal line, 4 tsun above the umbilicus.

ANATOMY: NERVE: 9th intercostal nerve.

MERIDIAN: Belongs to Jen-Mo.

INDICATIONS: Pain in the stomach region, abdominal distention, acid ructus, vomiting, constipation, diarrhea, indigestion, infantile ricketsia, madness, high blood pressure, neurasthenia, weakened body and hemoptysis.

10. KUAN-YUAN (JEN 4)

LOCATION: On the mid-abdominal line, 3 tsun below the umbilicus.

ANATOMY: NERVE: 12th intercostal nerve.

MERIDIAN: Belongs to Jen-Mo, and is the meeting point of the Leg Three Yin meridians and Jen-Mo.

INDICATIONS: Incontinence of urine, impotence, premature ejaculation, irregular menstruation, amenorrhea, lenkorrhagia, diarrhea, dysentery, nocturnal pollutions, blood in urine, frequent micturition, ascariasis.

11. CHUNG-CHI (JEN 3)

LOCATION: On the mid-abdominal line, 4 tsun below the umbilicus.

ANATOMY: NERVE: Branch of ilio-hypogastric arising from L1.

MERIDIAN: Belongs to Jen-Mo, and is the meeting point of the Leg three Yang meridians and Jen-Mo.

INDICATIONS: Impotence, premature ejaculation, irregular menstruation, incontinence of urine.

12. KUI-LAI (S 29)

LOCATION: 2 tsun beside the Chung-chi (Jen 3) point.

ANATOMY: NERVE: Branch of ilio-hypogastric arising from L1.

MERIDIAN: Belongs to the Arm Sunlight Yang (stomach) meridian.

INDICATIONS: Irregular menstruation, amenorrhea, leukorrhagia, disturbance of the intestine function, orchitis, prostatitis.

13. CHU-KU (JEN 2)

LOCATION: On the mid-abdominal line, 5 tsun below the umbilicus.

ANATOMY: NERVE: Branch of ilio-hypogastric arising from L1.

MERIDIAN: Belongs to Jen-Mo, is the meeting point of the Leg Absolute Yin (liver) meridian and Jen-Mo.

INDICATIONS: Urinary system and its diseases.

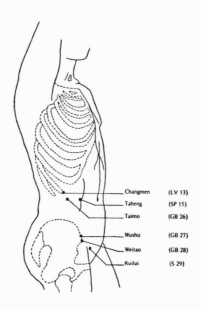

Changmen	(LV 13)
Taheng	(SP 15)
Taimo	(GB 26)
Wushu	(GB 27)
Weitao	(GB 28)
Kuilai	(S 29)

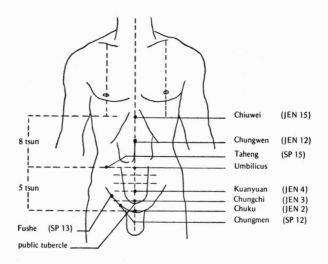

Chiuwei	(JEN 15)
Chungwen	(JEN 12)
Taheng	(SP 15)
Umbilicus	
Kuanyuan	(JEN 4)
Chungchi	(JEN 3)
Chuku	(JEN 2)
Chungmen	(SP 12)

8 tsun

5 tsun

Fushe   (SP 13)

public tubercle

FIGURE 54. *Acupuncture points on the abdomen.*

114

11

ACUPUNCTURE POINTS ON THE LUMBAR AND BACK REGION

See figures

1. CHIH-PIEN (B 49)

   LOCATION: Below the 4th spinous process of the sacral vertebra, 3 tsun beside the mid-dorsal line and also 1.5 tsun beside Pai-Huan-Shu.

   ANATOMY: MUSCLE: Greatest gluteal.

   NERVE: In the deep layer are: inferior gluteal nerve arising from L5, L5, S1 and S2, origin of the posterior cutaneous of the femoral nerve, sciatic nerve.

   MERIDIAN: Belongs to the Leg Great Tang (bladder) meridian.

   INDICATIONS: Palsy, lumbago, cystitis, sciatica, hemorrhoids.

2. CHUNG-LIAO (B 33)

   LOCATION: On the third posterior sacral foramen, at the antero-inferior part of Yzu-Liao.

   ANATOMY: MUSCLE: Origin of greatest gluteal.

   NERVE: Posterior branch of the 3rd sacral nerve.

115

MERIDIAN: Belongs to the Leg Greater Yang (bladder) meridian and is the meeting point of the Leg Absolute Yin (liver) and Leg Lesser Yang (gallbladder) meridians.

INDICATIONS: Orchitis, sciatica, unirosexual illness, hemorrhoids, uragogue, irregular menstruation.

3. TZU-LIAO (B 32)

LOCATION: On the second posterior sacral foramen and on the antero-inferior part of the postero-superior iliac spine.

ANATOMY: MUSCLE: Origin of greatest gluteal.

NERVE: Posterior branch of the 2nd sacral nerve.

MERIDIAN: Belongs to the Leg Greater Yang (bladder) meridian.

INDICATIONS: Same as No. 2.

4. SHANG-LIAO (B 31)

LOCATION: On the first posterior sacral foramen one tsun beside the mid-dorsal line and below the transversal process of the 5th lumbar vertebra.

ANATOMY: MUSCLE: Sacro-spinous and origin of greatest gluteal.

NERVE: Posterior branch of first sacral nerve.

MERIDIAN: Belongs to the Leg Greater Yang (bladder) meridian, and is the Lo point of the bladder and the Gallbladder meridian.

INDICATIONS: Same as No. 2.

5. PAI-HUAN-SHU (B 30)

LOCATION: Below the spinous process of the 4th sacral vertebra 1.5 tsun beside the mid-dorsal line.

ANATOMY: MUSCLE: Greatest gluteal.

NERVE: Cutaneous branch of infragluteal arising from S2 and S3. Nerve trunk formed by the lateral branches of the 1st, 2nd and 3rd sacral nerves.

MERIDIAN: Belongs to the Leg Greater Yang (bladder) meridian.

INDICATIONS: Infantile paralysis, endometritis, cramp in the circular muscle of anus, sciatica.

6. TA-CHANG-SHU (B 25)

LOCATION: Below the spinous process of the 4th lumbar vertebra, and 1.5 tsun beside the mid-dorsal line.

ANATOMY: MUSCLE: Superficial Layer: lumbo dorsal fascia. Deep layer: between the longus and iliocostal muscles.
NERVE: Posterior branch of 3rd lumbar nerve.

MERIDIAN: Belongs to the Leg Greater Yang (bladder) meridian.

INDICATIONS: Chronic diarrhea, lumbago, palsy of lower limb, infantile paralysis, sciatica, enteritis, constipation.

7. CHI-HAI-SHU (B 24)

LOCATION: Below the transversal process of the 3rd lumbar vetebra and 1 tsun beside the mid-dorsal line.

ANATOMY: MUSCLE: Superficial layer: lumbo dorsal fascia. Deep layer: between the longus and iliocostal muscles.
NERVE: Lateral cutaneous branch of the 2nd lumbar nerve, in the deep layer is the lateral cutaneous branch of the first lumbar nerve.

MERIDIAN: Belongs to the Leg Greater Yang (bladder) meridian.

INDICATIONS: Lumbago, hemorrhoids, weakness.

8. SHEN-SHU (B 23)

LOCATION: Below the spinous process of the second lumbar vertebra and 1.5 tsun beside the mid-dorsal line.

ANATOMY: MUSCLE: Superficial layer: lumbodorsal fascia. Deep layer: between the longus and iliocostal muscle.

NERVE: Lateral cutaneous branch of the first lumbar nerve; in the deep layer is the lateral branch of the first lumbar nerve.

MERIDIAN: Belongs to the Leg Greater Yang (bladder) meridian. Is Kidney point.

INDICATIONS: Nephritis, lumbago, neurasthenia, incontinence of urine, seminal emissions, impotence.

9. KAN-SHU (B 18)

LOCATION: Below the spinous process of the 9th thoracic vertebra and 1.5 tsun beside the mid-dorsal line.

ANATOMY: MUSCLE: Superficial layer: broadest part of back. Deep layer: Between the longus and iliocostal muscle.

NERVE: Medial branch of the 9th thoracic nerve. In the deep layer is the lateral branch of the 9th thoracic nerve.

MERIDIAN: Belongs to the Leg Greater Yang (bladder) meridian and is the Liver point.

INDICATIONS: Hepatitis, watery eyes, neurasthenia, intercostal neuralgia.

10. HSIN-SHU (B 15)

LOCATION: Below the spinous process of the 5th thoracic vertebra and 1.5 tsun beside the mid-dorsal line.

ANATOMY: MUSCLE: Supraspinous and interspinous ligaments.

NERVE: Medial branch of the 5th thoracic nerve.

MERIDIAN: Belongs to the Leg Greater Yang (bladder)

meridian and is the Heart point.

INDICATIONS: All kinds of heart disease, ulcer or hemorrhoid in the stomach region, vomiting, epilepsy.

11. FEI-SHU (B 13)

LOCATION: Below the spinous process of the 3rd thoracic vertebra and 1.5 tsun beside the mid-dorsal line.

ANATOMY: MUSCLE: Lumbodorsal fasciae. Supraspinous and interspinous ligaments.

NERVE: Medial branches of the 3rd thoracic nerve.

MERIDIAN: Belongs to the Leg Greater Yang (bladder) meridian and is the Lung point.

INDICATIONS: Chest discomfort, common colds, bronchitis, trachitis, tuberculosis of the lungs, itching.

12. CHIEN-CHUNG-SHU (SI 15)

LOCATION: 2 tsun beside the spinous process of the cervical vertebra.

ANATOMY: MUSCLE: Trapezius, levator of scapula.

NERVE: Lateral branch of first thoracic nerve, dorsal of scapula nerve arising from C5.

MERIDIAN: Belongs to the Arm Greater Yang (small intestine) meridian.

INDICATIONS: Backache, neckache, trachitis, asthma.

13. YAO-SHU (TU 2)

LOCATION: Below the 4th sacral vertebra, in the middle of the sacral hiatus.

ANATOMY: MUSCLE: Sacro-coccygeal ligament.

NERVE: Branch of the coccygeal nerve arising from S4-S5.

MERIDIAN: Belongs to Tu-Mo.

INDICATIONS: Infantile paralysis, palsy of lower limb, irregular menstruation, rectocele, lumbago.

14. YAO-YANG-KUAN (TU 3)

LOCATION: Between the spinous processes of the 4th and the 5th lumbar vertebrae, on the same level with the iliac crest.

ANATOMY: MUSCLE: Lumbodorsal fasciae, supraspinous ligament and interspinous ligament.
NERVE: Posterior branch of the 4th lumbar nerve.

MERIDIAN: Belongs to Tu-Mo.

INDICATIONS: Enteritis, lumbago, impotence, irregular menstruation, palsy of lower limb.

15. MING-MEN (TU 4)

LOCATION: Between the spinous processes of the second and third lumbar vertebrae.

ANATOMY: MUSCLE: Lumbodorsal fasciae. Supraspinous ligament and interspinous ligament.
NERVE: Posterior branch of the 2nd lumbar nerve.

MERIDIAN: Belongs to Yu-Mo.

INDICATIONS: Lumbago, diseases of urinary and generative system, endometritis, impotence, headache, tinnitus, prostatism or prostatitis.

16. SHEN-TAO (TU 11)

LOCATION: Between the spinous processes of the 5th and 6th thoracic vertebrae.

ANATOMY: MUSCLE: Lumbodorsal fasciae. Supraspinous and interspinous ligaments.
NERVE: Medial branch of the 5th thoracic nerve.

MERIDIAN: Belongs to Tu-Mo.

INDICATIONS: Neurasthenia, backache, cough, intercostal neuralgia, cholecystitis, lymphadenitis.

17. TAO-TAO (TU 13)

LOCATION: Between the spinous processes of the first and second thoracic vertebrae.

ANATOMY: MUSCLE: Lumbodorsal faciae. Supraspinous and interspinous ligaments.

NERVE: Medial branch of the 1st thoracic nerve.

MERIDIAN: Belongs to Tu-Mo and is the meeting point of the Leg Greater Yang (bladder) meridian and Tu-Mo.

INDICATIONS: Headache, dizziness, back and neck ache, asthma.

18. TA-CHUI (TU 14)

LOCATION: Between the spinous process of the 7th cervical vertebra and that of the first thoracic vertebra.

ANATOMY: MUSCLE: Lumbodorsal fasciae. Supraspinous and interspinous ligaments.

NERVE: Medial branches of the 8th cervical and first thoracic nerves.

MERIDIAN: Belongs to Tu-Mo and is the meeting point of the Leg Three Yang meridians, the Arm Three Yang meridians and Tu-Mo.

INDICATIONS: Asthma, common cold, fever, epilepsy, bronchitis, hepatitis, madness, psychogenesis.

19. TIN-CHUAN (Strange point)

LOCATION: 1 tsun beside Ta-Chui.

ANATOMY: same as No. 18.

MERIDIAN: Outside of the meridian.

INDICATIONS: Asthma, bronchitis.

20. HUA-TO'S VERTEBRAL POINTS (Strange point)

LOCATION: From below the spinous process of the first thoracic vertebra to below the spinous process of the 5th lumbar vertebra, each pair at a distance of ½ tsun beside the mid-dorsal line. There are 17 pairs or 34 Hua-To's Vertebral Points.

MERIDIAN: Outside of the meridian.

INDICATIONS: Asthma, diseases of the lung, diseases of gastro-intestinal tract, diseases of liver and gallbladder, disease of urinary and generative systems, lumbago, paralysis, neuralgia, weakness.

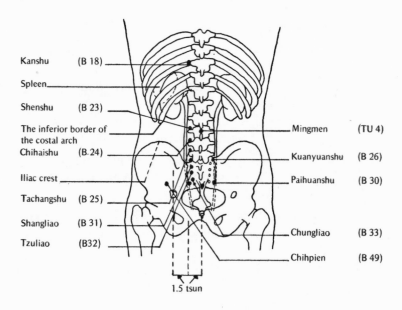

FIGURE 55. *Acupuncture points on the lumbo-sacral region.*

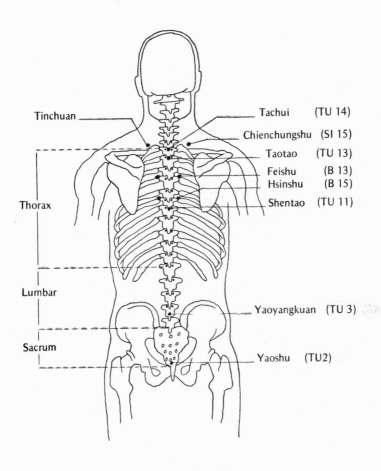

Tinchuan

Tachui   (TU 14)
Chienchungshu (SI 15)
Taotao   (TU 13)
Feishu   (B 13)
Hsinshu   (B 15)
Shentao   (TU 11)

Thorax

Lumbar

Yaoyangkuan   (TU 3)

Sacrum

Yaoshu   (TU2)

FIGURE 56. *Hua To's Vertebral Points.*

12

ACUPUNCTURE POINTS ON THE UPPER LIMB

See figures

1. YUN-MEN (L 2)

   LOCATION: In the infraclavicular fossa.

   ANATOMY: MUSCLE: Greater pectoral, deltoid.
   NERVE: Arising from the C3–T1 segments. Superficial layer: medial and posterior branches of the superior clavicular nerve. Deep layer: branches of anterior thoracic nerve and lateral fasciculus of the brachial plexus.

   MERIDIAN: Belongs to the Arm Greater Yin (lungs) meridian.

   INDICATIONS: Asthma, cough, stridor, frozen shoulder, pain in the shoulder blade, backache, pain in the chest.

2. CHIH-TSE (L 5)

   LOCATION: At the elbow crease on the lateral border of the tendon of the biceps brachii muscle.

   ANATOMY: MUSCLE: Radial side of the tendon of the biceps brachii.
   NERVE: Arising from C5–T1: in the superficial layer is the lateral antebrachial cutaneous; in the deep layer is the radial nerve.

   MERIDIAN: Belongs to the Arm Greater Yin (lungs) meridian.

INDICATIONS: Asthma, cough, pharyngitis, hemoptysis, pain in the elbow.

3. KUNG-TSUI (L 6)

LOCATION: 7 tsun above the most distal skin crease of the wrist on the radial side of the anterior surface of the forearm.

ANATOMY: MUSCLE: Brachioradial, long and short radial extensors of wrist.

NERVE: Arising from C5–T1: in the superficial layer is the lateral antebrachial cutaneous; in the deep layer is the radial nerve.

MERIDIAN: Belongs to the Arm Greater Yin (lungs) meridian.

INDICATIONS: Asthma, cough, hemoptysis, tonsillitis, arm pains.

4. LIEH-CHUEH (L 7)

LOCATION: 1.5 tsun above the most distal skin crease of the wrist, above the styloid process of the radius.

ANATOMY: MUSCLE: Between tendon of brachioradial and tendon of the long abductor of thumb.

NERVE: Arising from C5–T1: in the superficial layer is lateral antebrachial cutaneous; in the deep layer is the superficial branch of radial nerve.

MERIDIAN: Belongs to Arm Greater Yin (lungs) meridian.

INDICATIONS: Headache, vertigo, cough, facial nerve paralysis, asthma, neckache.

5. YU-CHI (L 10)

LOCATION: On the palmar surface at the middle of the first metacarpal bone.

ANATOMY: MUSCLE: Short abductor and adductor of thumb.

NERVE: Lateral antebrachial cutaneous nerve arising from C5–T1 and superficial branches of radial nerve.

MERIDIAN: Belongs to Arm Greater Yin (lungs) meridian.

INDICATIONS: Asthma, cough, hemoptysis, pharyngitis.

6. HSI-MEN (HC 4)

LOCATION: 5 tsun above the most distal skin crease of the wrist in front of the forearm.

ANATOMY: MUSCLE: Between radial flexor of wrist and long palmar, superficial flexor of fingers, deep flexor of fingers.
NERVE: Arising from C6–T1 Superficial layer: medial antebrachial cutaneous. Deep layer: median nerve. Deepest layer: volar interosseus.

MERIDIAN: Belongs to the Arm Absolute Yin (heart constrictor) meridian.

INDICATIONS: Palpitation, angina pectoris, irritable heart, neurasthenia.

7. NEI-KUAN (HC 6)

LOCATION: 2 tsun above the most distal skin crease of the wrist in front of the forearm.

ANATOMY: MUSCLE: Between radial flexor of wrist and long palmar, superficial and deep flexors of fingers.
NERVE: Arising from C6–T1. In the superficial layer: medial antebrachial cutaneous. In the deep layer: median nerve. In the deepest layer: volar interosseus.

MERIDIAN: Belongs to the Arm Absolute Yin (heart constrictor) meridian separated into the Arm Lesser Yang (triple heater) meridian, and is one point passed by Yang-Wei-Mo.

INDICATIONS: Chest pain, cardial colic, vomiting, mental anomaly, hysteria.

8. CHING-LING (H 2)

LOCATION: 3 tsun above the medial side of the elbow crease at the medial side of the tendons of the biceps brachii muscle.

ANATOMY: MUSCLE: Triceps brachii.

NERVE: Ulnar nerve arising from C8–T1. Medial antebrachial cutaneous and medial brachial cutaneous.

MERIDIAN: Belongs to the Arm Lesser Yin (heart) meridian.

INDICATIONS: Pain in the shoulder joints, arm pains, intercostal pain.

9. SHAO-HAI (H 3)

LOCATION: At the medial side of the elbow crease when the elbow is flexed.

ANATOMY: MUSCLE: Round pronator, brachial muscles.

NERVE: Medial antebrachial cutaneous arising from C5–T1.

MERIDIAN: Belongs to Arm Lesser Yin (heart) meridian.

INDICATIONS: Chest pain, intercostal pain, ulnar pain.

10. TUNG-LI (H 5)

LOCATION: 1 tsun above the most distal skin crease of the wrist on the ulnar side in the front of the forearm.

ANATOMY: MUSCLE: Between the tendon of ulnar flexor of wrist and superficial flexor of fingers and in the deep layer is the deep flexor of fingers.

NERVE: Medial antebrachial cutaneous arising from L8–T1; ulnar nerve.

MERIDIAN: Belongs to the Arm Lesser Yin (heart) meridian, separated into the Arm Greater Yang (small intestine) meridian.

INDICATIONS: Hysteria, neurasthenia, chest pain, angina pectoris.

11. ERH-CHIEN (LI 2)

LOCATION: On the dorsum of the hand, at the radial side of the proximal end of the index finger when the fist is slightly closed.

ANATOMY: MUSCLE: Deep and superficial tendon of flexor of the fingers.

NERVE: Arising from C5–T1. Branch of the proper volar digital of median nerve and branch of dorsal digital.

MERIDIAN: Belongs to the Arm Sunlight Yang (large intestine) meridian, and is the point on the radial nerve.

INDICATIONS: Facial nerve paralysis, toothache, pharyngis, backache, epistaxis.

12. SAN-CHIEN (LI 3)

LOCATION: On the dorsum of the hand, above the radial side of the distal part of the 2nd metacarpal bone.

ANATOMY: MUSCLE: Dorsal interosseus and adductor of thumb.

NERVE: Superficial branch of radial nerve arising from C5–T1.

MERIDIAN: Belongs to the Arm Sunlight Yang (large intestine) meridian.

INDICATIONS: Eye pain, tooth pain, trifacial nerve pain.

13. HO-KU (LI 4)

LOCATION: On the dorsum of the hand, between the first and the second radial side in the middle of the 2nd metacarpal bone.

ANATOMY: MUSCLE: First dorsal interosseus and adductor of thumb.

NERVE: Arising from C5–T1. Branch of radial nerve on dorsal side of the hand and branch of the proper volar digital of median nerve.

MERIDIAN: Belongs to Arm Sunlight Yan (large intestine) meridian.

INDICATIONS: Headache, epistaxis, laryngophargitis, facial nerve paralysis, toothache.

14. CHU-CHIH (LI 11)

LOCATION: At the external end of the elbow crease when the elbow is flexed.

ANATOMY: MUSCLE: Origin of long radial extensor of wrist.

NERVE: Arising from C5–T1. Superficial layer: antebrachial cutaneous branch of radial nerve. Deep layer: the radial nerve.

MERIDIAN: Belongs to the Arm Sunlight Yang (large intestine) meridian.

INDICATIONS: Pain in the shoulders and arms, hemiplegia, tonsillitis, fever, high blood pressure, skin disease, lymphocele, painful oropharynx, goiter, jumping disease.

15. PI-NAO (LI 14)

LOCATION: 7 tsun above chu-chih at the insertion of the deltoid muscle.

ANATOMY: MUSCLE: Posterior margin of insertion of deltoid and anterolateral margin of triceps brachii.

NERVE: Arising from C5–T1. Superficial layer: the dorsalbrachial cutaneous. Deep layer: the radial nerve.

MERIDIAN: Belongs to the Arm Sunlight Yang (large intestine) meridian and is the meeting point of the Arm Sunlight Yang (large intestine) meridian and Lo-Mo and Yang-Wei-Mo.

INDICATIONS: Chest pain, backache, arm pains, shoulder pains, hemiplegia, eye diseases.

16. CHIEN-YU (LI 15)

LOCATION: At the antero-inferior point of the acromion, where a depression is formed when the arm is raised.

ANATOMY: MUSCLE: Upper part of deltoid.

NERVE: Arising from C4–T1. Supra clavicular and axillar nerves.

MERIDIAN: Belongs to the Arm Sunlight Yang (large intestine) meridian and is the meeting point of the Arm Sunlight Yang (large intestine) meridian and Yang-Chiao-Mo.

INDICATIONS: Hemiplegia, paralysis of upper limb, locomotor disturbance, pain in the shoulder joints.

17. CHUNG-CHU (TH 3)

LOCATION: Between the 4th and 5th metacarpal bones, and 1 tsun above the web of the fingers.

ANATOMY: MUSCLE: Fourth interosseus.

NERVE: Arising from C8–T1. Branch of ulnar nerve on dorsal side of hand.

MERIDIAN: Belongs to the Arm Lesser Yang (triple heater) meridian.

INDICATIONS: Deafness, dumbness, tinnitus, shoulder and back pain.

18. WAI-KUAN (TH 5)

LOCATION: 2 tsun above the skin crease on the back of the wrist between the ulnar and radius.

ANATOMY: MUSCLE: Between long extensor of thumb and common extensor of fingers.

NERVE: Arising from C5–T1. Superficial layer is the dorsal antebrachial cutaneous. Deep layer is the dorsal antebrachial interosseus.

MERIDIAN: Belongs to the Arm Lesser Yang (triple heater) meridian and separated into the Arm Absolute Yang (heart constrictor) meridian and also passed by Yang-Wei-Mo

INDICATIONS: Parotitis, neuralgia of forearm, arthritis of the upper limb, neck pain, deafness, dumbness, hemiplegia.

19. CHIH-KOU (TH 6)

LOCATION: 3 tsun above the skin crease of the back of the wrist between the ulnar and radius.

ANATOMY: MUSCLE: Between long extensor of thumb and common extensor of fingers.

NERVE: Arising from C5–T1. In the superficial layer is the dorsal antebrachial cutaneous. In the deep layer is the dorsal antebrachial interosseus.

MERIDIAN: Belongs to the Arm Lesser Yang (triple heater) meridian.

INDICATIONS: Shoulder or arm pains, constipation, deafness.

20. SAN-YANG-LO (TH 8)

LOCATION: 1 tsun above Chih-Kou.

ANATOMY: MUSCLE: Common extensor of fingers.

NERVE: Arising from C5–T1. In the superficial layer is the dorsal antebrachial cutaneous. In the deep layer is the dorsal antebrachial interosseus.

MERIDIAN: Belongs to the Arm Lesser Yang (triple heater) meridian.

INDICATIONS: Deafness, dumbness, arm pains.

21. NAO-HUI (TH 13)

LOCATION: 3 tsun from the acromion, just below the deltoid muscle.

ANATOMY: MUSCLE: In the middle of triceps brachii.

NERVE: Arising from C6–T1. Radial nerve and dorsal brachial cutaneous.

MERIDIAN: Belongs to the Arm Lesser Yang (triple heater) meridian. Joining point of the Arm Lesser Yang (triple heater) meridian and Yang-Wei-Mo.

INDICATIONS: Shoulder and arm pains.

22. HOU-HSI (SI 3)

LOCATION: Laterally behind the distal end of 5th metacarpal bone when the fist is slightly clenched.

ANATOMY: MUSCLE: Abductor of 5th finger.
NERVE: Volar and dorsal branches of ulnar nerve arising from C7–T1.

MERIDIAN: Belongs to the Arm Greater Yang (small intestine) meridian and passed by Yu-Mo.

INDICATIONS: Deafness, dumbness, headache, backache, lumbago, intercostal neuralgia.

23. YANG-LAO (SI 6)

LOCATION: On the radial side of the distal head of the ulna, with the palm of the hand facing the breast.

ANATOMY: MUSCLE: Between the tendon of ulnar extensor of wrist end tendon of extensor of the 5th finger.
NERVE: Arising from C5–T1. Dorsal antebrachial cutaneous and volar and dorsal branches of ulnar nerve.

MERIDIAN: Belongs to the Arm Greater Yang (small intestine) meridian.

INDICATIONS: Arthritis of upper limb, hysteria, neuralgia of head-back (Occiput), shoulder pains.

24. CHIEN-CHENG (SI 9)

LOCATION: 1 tsun above the posterior axillary fold at the

inferoposterior part of the shoulder joint.

ANATOMY: MUSCLE: Posterior margin of deltoid. In the deep layer is the large long muscle.

NERVE: Arising from C5–T1. Branches of axillary and radial nerve.

MERIDIAN: Belongs to the Arm Greater Yang (small intestine) meridian.

INDICATIONS: Shoulder pain, arm cannot be raised, tinnitus, deafness.

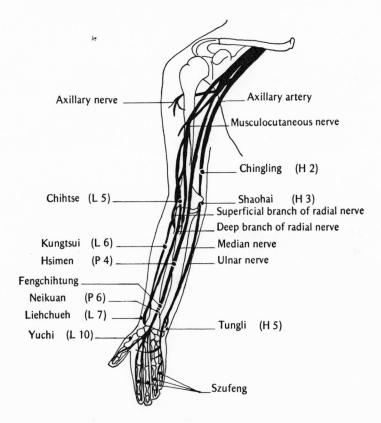

FIGURE 57. *Relation between acupuncture points on the anterior surface of the upper limb and the nerves.*

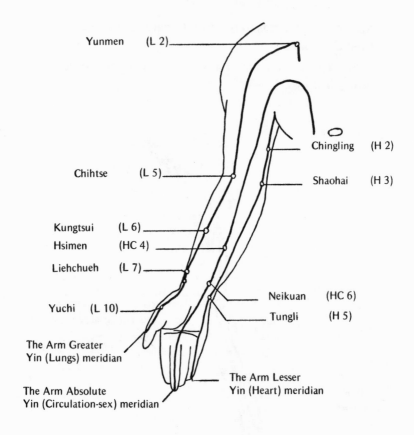

Yunmen   (L 2)

Chingling   (H 2)

Chihtse   (L 5)

Shaohai   (H 3)

Kungtsui   (L 6)
Hsimen   (HC 4)

Liehchueh   (L 7)

Neikuan   (HC 6)

Yuchi   (L 10)

Tungli   (H 5)

The Arm Greater
Yin (Lungs) meridian

The Arm Lesser
Yin (Heart) meridian

The Arm Absolute
Yin (Circulation-sex) meridian

FIGURE 58. *Acupuncture points on the anterior surface of the upper limb.*

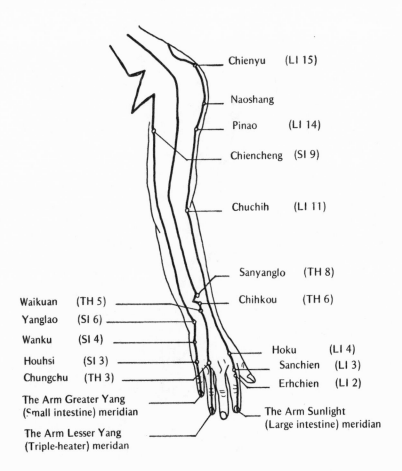

Chienyu   (LI 15)

Naoshang

Pinao   (LI 14)

Chiencheng   (SI 9)

Chuchih   (LI 11)

Sanyanglo   (TH 8)

Waikuan   (TH 5)
Yanglao   (SI 6)
Wanku   (SI 4)

Chihkou   (TH 6)

Houhsi   (SI 3)
Chungchu   (TH 3)

Hoku   (LI 4)
Sanchien   (LI 3)
Erhchien   (LI 2)

The Arm Greater Yang
(Small intestine) meridian

The Arm Lesser Yang
(Triple-heater) meridan

The Arm Sunlight
(Large intestine) meridian

FIGURE 59. *Acupuncture points on the posterior surface of the upper limb.*

135

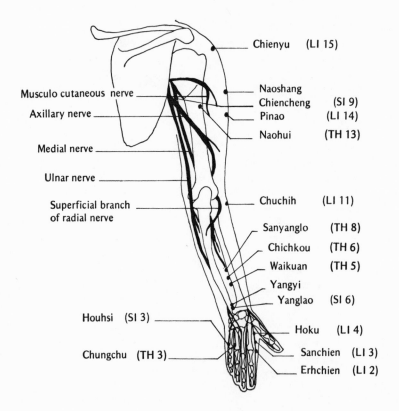

Chienyu   (LI 15)

Musculo cutaneous nerve

Naoshang

Chiencheng   (SI 9)

Axillary nerve

Pinao   (LI 14)

Naohui   (TH 13)

Medial nerve

Ulnar nerve

Superficial branch
of radial nerve

Chuchih   (LI 11)

Sanyanglo   (TH 8)

Chichkou   (TH 6)

Waikuan   (TH 5)

Yangyi

Yanglao   (SI 6)

Houhsi   (SI 3)

Chungchu   (TH 3)

Hoku   (LI 4)

Sanchien   (LI 3)

Erhchien   (LI 2)

FIGURE 60. *Relation between acupuncture points on the posterior surface of the upper limb and the nerves.*
136

13

ACUPUNCTURE POINTS ON THE HEAD, FACE, NECK AND NAPE REGIONS

See figures

1. YING-HSIANG (LI 20)

   LOCATION: ½ tsun beside the ala nasi, in the nasolabial sulcus.

   ANATOMY: MUSCLE: Quadrate muscle of upper lip.
   NERVE: Anastomosis of facial nerve with the infraorbital branch of trigeminus.

   MERIDIAN: Belongs to the Arm Sunlight Yang (large intestine) meridian, is the meeting point of the Arm Sunlight Yang (large intestine) and the Leg Sunlight Yang (stomach) meridians.

   INDICATIONS: Rhinitis, nasosinusitis, facial nerve paralysis, pain in the stomach region.

2. FU-TU (LI 18)

   LOCATION: On the lateral side of the neck region, in the middle of the posterior margin of sternocleidomastoid muscle.

   ANATOMY: MUSCLE: Splenius, sternocleidomastoid, in the deep layer is the origin of levator of the shoulder blade.
   NERVE: Great auricular nerve arising from C II–C V. Cutaneus of cervical nerve, smaller occipital nerve.

137

MERIDIAN: Belongs to the Arm Sunlight Yang (large intestine) meridian.

INDICATIONS: Sore-throat, asthma, expectoration.

3. CHUAN-LIAO (SI 18)

LOCATION: Directly below the external canthus on the lower border of the zygomatic bone at the same level of Ying-Hsiang.

ANATOMY: MUSCLE: Origin of masseter, in the middle of zygomaticus.

NERVE: Facial nerve and infraorbital branch of trigeminus.

MERIDIAN: Belongs to the Arm Greater Yang (small intestine) meridian and is the meeting point of the Arm Greater Yang (small intestine) and the Arm Lesser Yang (triple heater) meridian.

INDICATIONS: Facial nerve analysis, toothache.

4. CHENG-CHI (S 1)

LOCATION: 7 fen (10 fen equal 1 tsun) just below the pupil, between the eyeball and the inferior border of the orbit, with the eyes looking straight ahead.

ANATOMY: MUSCLE: Orbicular of eye, in the orbita are the inferior rectus and inferior oblique of the eyeball.

NERVE: Orbital branch of trigeminus, oculomotor, branch of facial nerve.

MERIDIAN: Belongs to the Leg Sunlight Yang (stomach) meridian and is the meeting point of the Leg Sunlight Yang (stomach) meridian, Yang-Chiao-Mo and Jen-Mo.

INDICATIONS: Myopia, neuralgia of the inferior orbit, conjunctivitis.

5. SZU-PAI (S 2)

LOCATION: At the depression over the infraorbital foramen.

ANATOMY: MUSCLE: Between Orbicular of eye and quadrate muscle of upper lip.
NERVE: Branch of facial and infraorbital branch of trigeminus.

MERIDIAN: Belongs to the Leg Sunlight Yang (stomach) meridian.

INDICATIONS: Myopia, facial nerve spasm or paralysis, anaphylactic swollen face.

6. CHU-LIAO (S 3)

LOCATION: Directly below Szu-pai, at the level with the inferior border of the ala nasi.

ANATOMY: MUSCLE: Superficial layer: quadrate muscle of upper lip. Deep layer: canine muscle.
NERVE: Near facial, infraorbital branch of trigeminus.

MERIDIAN: Belongs to the Leg Sunlight Yang (stomach) meridian, the meeting point of Leg Sunlight Yang (stomach) meridian and Yang-Chiao-Mo.

INDICATIONS: Facial nerve paralysis, toothache, epistaxis, cheek pain.

7. HSIA-KUAN (S 7)

LOCATION: About 1 tsun in front of the tragus, in the depression between the inferior border of the zygomatic arch and the mandibular arch.

ANATOMY: MUSCLE: Origin of masseter.
NERVE: Zygomatico-orbital branch and auriculo temporal branch of facial nerve, in the deep layer is the mandibular branch of the trigeminus nerve.

MERIDIAN: Belongs to the Leg Sunlight Yang (stomach)

meridian and is the meeting point of the Leg Sunlight Yang (stomach) meridian and the Leg Lesser Yang (gallbladder) meridian.

INDICATIONS: Toothache, arthritis of the mandible, trismus, facial nerve paralysis.

8. CHIA-CHE (S 6)

LOCATION: About 1 tsun at the supero-anterior part of the angle of the mandible.

ANATOMY: MUSCLE: Masseter.
NERVE: Branches of facial and trigeminus, passed by the great auricular arising from C3–C5.

MERIDIAN: Belongs to the Leg Sunlight Yang (stomach) meridian.

INDICATIONS: Toothache, arthritis of the mandible, facial nerve paralysis, parotitis.

9. TA-YING (S 5)

LOCATION: In front of the angle of the mandible on the anterior border of the masseter muscle.

ANATOMY: MUSCLE: Anterior margin of end of masseter.
NERVE: Branches of trigeminus and facial nerve.

MERIDIAN: Belongs to the Leg Sunlight Yang (stomach) meridian.

INDICATIONS: Facial muscle spasm, facial nerve paralysis, toothache, parotitis, stomatitis.

10. TING-HUI (GB 2)

LOCATION: Below erhmen in front of the incisura intertragicia where a depression is formed when the mouth is wide open.

ANATOMY: MUSCLE: Ear.

NERVE: Great auricular arising from C2 and C3.

MERIDIAN: Belongs to the Leg Lesser Yang (gallbladder) meridian.

INDICATIONS: Deafness, tinnitus aurium, deaf-mutism, otitis media, facial nerve paralysis.

11. SHUAI-KU (GB 8)

LOCATION: Above the apex of the auricular and 1.5 tsun above the natural line of the hair.

ANATOMY: MUSCLE: Temporal.

NERVE: Joining point of the temporal nerve originating from C2 and C3 and occipital nerve.

MERIDIAN: Belongs to the Leg Lesser Yang (gallbladder) meridian and is the meeting point of the Leg Lesser Yang (gallbladder) and Leg Greater Yang (bladder) meridian.

INDICATIONS: Megrim.

12. YANG-PAI (GB 14)

LOCATION: 1 tsun above the middle of the eyebrow, in the depression on the superciliary arch.

ANATOMY: MUSCLE: Frontal.

NERVE: Supra orbital branch of trigeminus.

MERIDIAN: Belongs to the Leg Lesser Yang (gallbladder) meridian and is the meeting point of the Arm Lesser Yang (triple heater), the Leg Lesser Yang (gallbladder) and Arm Sunlight Yang (large intestine) meridian and the meeting point of the Leg Sunlight Yang (stomach) meridian and Yang-Wei-Mo.

INDICATIONS: Facial nerve paralysis, tremor of the eyes, pruritus and pain in the eyes, trigeminal neuralgia, orbital neuralgia.

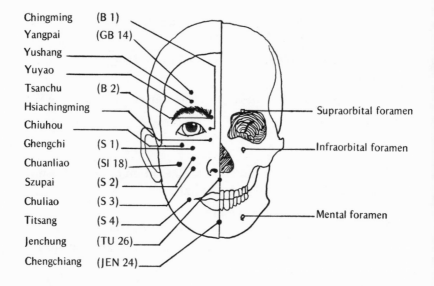

Chingming	(B 1)
Yangpai	(GB 14)
Yushang	
Yuyao	
Tsanchu	(B 2)
Hsiachingming	
Chiuhou	
Ghengchi	(S 1)
Chuanliao	(SI 18)
Szupai	(S 2)
Chuliao	(S 3)
Titsang	(S 4)
Jenchung	(TU 26)
Chengchiang	(JEN 24)

Supraorbital foramen

Infraorbital foramen

Mental foramen

FIGURE 61. *Acupuncture points on the face region.*

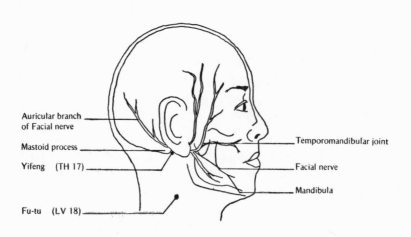

Auricular branch
of Facial nerve

Mastoid process

Yifeng   (TH 17)

Fu-tu   (LV 18)

Temporomandibular joint

Facial nerve

Mandibula

FIGURE 62. *Acupuncture points on the ear region and facial nerve.*
142

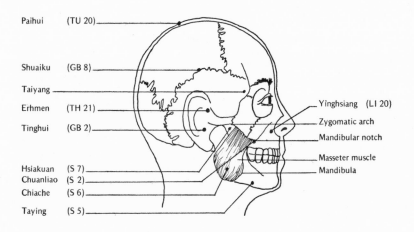

Paihui	(TU 20)	
Shuaiku	(GB 8)	
Taiyang		
Erhmen	(TH 21)	
Tinghui	(GB 2)	
Hsiakuan	(S 7)	
Chuanliao	(S 2)	
Chiache	(S 6)	
Taying	(S 5)	

Yinghsiang (LI 20)
Zygomatic arch
Mandibular notch
Masseter muscle
Mandibula

FIGURE 63. *Acupuncture points on the temporal and cheek regions.*

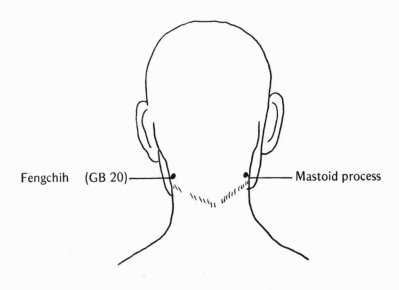

Fengchih (GB 20) ——— Mastoid process

FIGURE 64. *Acupuncture points on the upperneck region.*

143

13. FENG-CHIH (GB 20)

LOCATION: Behind the mastoid process on the outer part of the trapezius muscle, on a level with the ear lobe.

ANATOMY: MUSCLE: End of sternocleidomastoid and trapezius, in the deep layer is the captitus muscle. NERVE: Smaller occipital originating from C2-C5.

MERIDIAN: Belongs to the Leg Lesser Yang (gallbladder) meridian and is the meeting point of the Leg Lesser Yang (gallbladder) meridian and Yang-Wei-Mo.

INDICATIONS: Pain in the occiput, vertigo, eye disease, common cold, tinnitus aurium, facial nerve spasm.

14. CHING-MING (B 1)

LOCATION: On the border of the orbit and one fen below the inner canthus.

ANATOMY: MUSCLE: The middle of the medial palpebral ligament in the medial border of the orbit, in the deep layer is the medial rectus of the eye. NERVE: Infra and supra trochlear, ophthalmic and naso-ciliary nerve.

MERIDIAN: Belongs to the Leg Greater Yang (bladder) meridian and is the meeting point of the Arm and Leg Greater Yang, the Leg Sunlight Yang, Yang-Chiao-Mo and Yin-Chiao-Mo.

INDICATIONS: Tearing, night blindness, optic neuritis, rhinitis, optic nerve atrophy, cataract.

15. TSAN-CHU (B 2)

LOCATION: In the depression at the medial end of the eyebrow.

ANATOMY: MUSCLE: In the middle of the frontal and muscle corrugator glabellae. NERVE: Branch of the trigeminus, supratrochlear.

MERIDIAN: Belongs to the Leg Greater Yang (bladder) meridian.

INDICATIONS: Forehead neuralgia, tears, facial palsy.

16. JEN-CHUNG (TU 26)

LOCATION: Just above the middle of the philtrum.

ANATOMY: MUSCLE: Orbicular of mouth.
NERVE: Infraorbicular branch of trigeminus and branch of facial nerve for the cheek muscle.

MERIDIAN: Belongs to Tu-Mo and is the meeting point of Tu-Mo, the Leg Sunlight Yang (stomach) and the Arm Sunlight Yang (large intestine) meridians.

INDICATIONS: Shock, lumbago, stroke, unconsciousness.

17. PAI-HUI (TU 20)

LOCATION: 7 tsun from the middle of the natural line of hair.

ANATOMY: MUSCLE: Galea aponeurotica.
NERVE: Branch of the occipital nerve arising from C2.

MERIDIAN: Belongs to Tu-Mo, and is the meeting point of the Arm and Leg Yang meridians and Yu-Mo.

INDICATIONS: Shock, prolapse of anus, headache, vertigo, insomnia.

18. CHENG-CHIANG (JEN 24)

LOCATION: Middle of the depression of the mentolabial sulcus.

ANATOMY: MUSCLE: In the middle between quadrate muscle of lower lip and cheek muscle.
NERVE: Branch of the facial nerve.

MERIDIAN: Belongs to Jen-Mo and is the meeting point of

Jen-Mo and the Leg Sunlight Yang (stomach) meridian.

INDICATIONS: Facial paralysis, toothache, salivation, pain in the back neck.

19. ERH-MEN (TH 21)

LOCATION: In the front of the tuberculum supratragicum where a depression is formed when the mouth is opened

ANATOMY: NERVE: Auriculotemporal branch of facial nerve.

MERIDIAN: Belongs to the Arm Lesser Yang (triple heater) meridian.

INDICATIONS: Deafness, tinnitus, otitis media, toothache.

20. YI-FENG (TH 17)

LOCATION: Behind the lobule of the auricle, between the mastoid process and the mandible where a depression is formed, when the mouth is opened.

ANATOMY: NERVE: Facial nerve and great auricular arising from C2–C5.

MERIDIAN: Belongs to the Arm Lesser Yang (triple heater) meridian. Joining point of the triple heater meridian and the gallbladder meridian.

INDICATIONS: Deafness, tinnitus, facial nerve paralysis.

21. YU-YAO (Strange point)

LOCATION: Directly above the pupil in the middle of the eyebrow.

ANATOMY: MUSCLE: Origin of frontal and orbicular.
NERVE: Supraorbital branch of trigeminus.

MERIDIAN: Outside the meridian.

INDICATIONS: Rhinitis, optic muscle paralysis, inflammation of cornea.

22. YU-SHANG (Strange point)

LOCATION: Directly above Yu-yao, at the upper margin of

the middle of the eyebrow.

ANATOMY: MUSCLE: Orbicular of eye.

NERVE: Supraorbital branch of trigeminus.

MERIDIAN: Outside the meridian.

INDICATIONS: Same as Yu-yao.

23. HSIA-CHING-MING (Strange point)

LOCATION: On both sides of the nasal root in the medial border of the orbit.

ANATOMY: MUSCLE: In the deep layer is the medial rectus of the eye.

NERVE: Branch of oculomotor, branch of trigeminus passed by the supra and infratrochlear nerve.

MERIDIAN: Outside the meridian.

INDICATIONS: Night blindness, tears, optic neuritis, optic nerve atrophy, myopia.

24. TAI-YANG (Strange point)

LOCATION: In the depression, about 1 tsun lateral to the external canthus.

ANATOMY: NERVE: Auriculotemporal branch of trigeminus.

MERIDIAN: Outside the meridian.

INDICATIONS: Headache, diseases of the eye.

25. CHIU-HOU (Strange point)

LOCATION: At the inferior border of the orbit.

ANATOMY: MUSCLE: Orbicular of eye.

NERVE: Infraorbital branch of trigeminus, branch of oculomotor, branch of facial nerve.

MERIDIAN: Outside the meridian.

INDICATIONS: All kinds of eye disease, facial paralysis, neuralgia of the inferior orbit, conjunctivitis.

14

ACUPUNCTURE POINTS ON THE LOWER LIMB

See figures

1. PI-KUAN (S 31)

   LOCATION: Directly below the antero-superior spine of the ilium, on the lateral side of the sartorius muscle and at the same level with Hui-Yang (B 35).

   ANATOMY: MUSCLE: Between sartorius and tensor of broad fasciae.
   NERVE: Lateral femoral cutaneous arising from L2 and L3.

   MERIDIAN: Belongs to the Leg Sunlight Yang (stomach) meridian.

   INDICATIONS: Paralysis in the lower limb, palsy, lymphadenitis, lumbago.

2. TSU-SAN-LI (S 36)

   LOCATION: 3 tsun below the tuberosity of the tibia on the lateral side of the tibialis anterior muscle.

   ANATOMY: MUSCLE: Between anterior tibial and long extensor of toes.
   NERVE: Arising from L4–S1. Superficial layer: lateral sural cutaneous and the cutaneous branch of saphenous. Deep layer: the deep peroneal.

MERIDIAN: Belongs to the Leg Sunlight Yang (stomach) meridian.

INDICATIONS: Pain in the lower limb, palsy, abdominal pain, abdominal distention, constipation, diarrhea, vomiting, lumbago, skin disease, insomnia, infantile indigestion, larynx pain, epilepsy, anemia, jaundice, high blood pressure, hysteria, neurasthenia, gastritis, ulcer, gastroptosis.

3. SHANG-CHU-HSU (S 37)

LOCATION: 6 tsun below tupi, on the lateral side of the tibia.

ANATOMY: MUSCLE: Anterior tibial.
NERVE: Arising from L5–S1. Superficial layer: lateral sural cutaneous. Deep layer: deep paroneal.

MERIDIAN: Belongs to the Leg Sunlight Yang (stomach) meridian.

INDICATIONS: Abdominal pain, ascites, diarrhea, hysteria.

4. FENG-LUNG (S 40)

LOCATION: 8 tsun above the anterior part of the lateral malleolus, and 2 tsun lateral to the anterior margin of tibia.

ANATOMY: MUSCLE: Between lateral long extensor of toes and short peroneal.
NERVE: Superficial peroneal arising from L5–S1.

MERIDIAN: Belongs to the Leg Sunlight Yang (stomach) meridian, separated into the spleen meridian.

INDICATIONS: Abdominal pain, pain in the lower limb, mucous cough, vomiting, vertigo, headache, swollen and painful orpharynx, sputum.

5. CHIEH-HSI (S 41)

LOCATION: Over the dorsum of the foot right in the middle of the cruciate crural ligament.

ANATOMY: MUSCLE: Between tendon of long extensor of great toe and tendon of long extensor of toes. NERVE: Arising from L4–S1. Superficial layer: superficial peroneal. Deep layer: deep peroneal.

MERIDIAN: Belongs to the Leg Sunlight Yang (stomach) meridian.

INDICATIONS: Headache, arthritis in the ankle joints.

6. HSIEN-KU (S 43)

LOCATION: Between the 2nd and the 3rd metatarsal bones.

ANATOMY: MUSCLE: 2nd and 3rd interosseal. NERVE: Arising from L5–S1. Second medial cutaneous of superficial peroneal.

MERIDIAN: Belongs to the Leg Sunlight Yang (stomach) meridian.

INDICATIONS: Hydropsy, swelling in dorsum pedis.

7. NEI-TING (S 44)

LOCATION: ½ tsun behind the web between 2nd and 3rd toes.

ANATOMY: NERVE: Arising from L5–S1. On the place where the 2nd branch of the medial cutaneous of the dorsum of the foot sends off the dorsal nerve of the foot.

MERIDIAN: Belongs to the Leg Sunlight Yang (stomach) meridian.

INDICATIONS: Stomach pain, headache, toothache, tonsillitis, dysentery.

8. HUAN-TIAO (GB 30)

LOCATION: On the postero-superior side of the greater trochanter, ⅓ the distance, posteriorly, from the greater trochanter to the sacral hiatus.

ANATOMY: MUSCLE: Greatest gluteal.

NERVE: Arising from L4–S1. Superficial layer: the inferior gluteal cutaneous. Deep layer: the sciatic nerve.

MERIDIAN: Belongs to the Leg Lesser Yang (gallbladder) meridian and is the meeting point of the gallbladder meridian and the bladder meridian.

INDICATIONS: Pain in the loin and legs, sciatica, hemiplegia, paralysis of the lower limb, infantile paralysis.

9. FENG-SHIH (GB 31)

LOCATION: On the lateral part of the thigh, 7 tsun above the patella.

ANATOMY: MUSCLE: Lateral femoral and broad fasciae.

Nerve: Arising from T12–L3. Superficial layer: lateral femoral cutaneous. Deep layer: muscular branch of femoral nerve.

MERIDIAN: Belongs to the Leg Lesser Yang (gallbladder) meridian.

INDICATIONS: Hemiplegia, sciatica, arthritis of knees, infantile paralysis.

10. YANG-LING-CHUAN (GB 34)

LOCATION: On the antero-inferior part of the capitulum of the fibula, 2 tsun below the knee.

ANATOMY: MUSCLE: Long and short peroneal.

NERVE: Arising from L5-S1, in the place where the common peroneal divides into superficial and deep peroneal.

MERIDIAN: Belongs to the Leg Lesser Yang (gallbladder) meridian.

INDICATIONS: Pain in the lower limb, spasms or pain in the loins and legs, numbness, hemiplegia, high blood pressure, habitual constipation.

11. WAI-CHIU (GB 36)

LOCATION: 7 tsun above the lateral malleolus, in front of the fibula.

ANATOMY: MUSCLE: Long peroneal.
NERVE: Arising from L4–S1. Superficial layer: superficial peroneal lateral sural cutaneous. Deep layer: deep peroneal.

MERIDIAN: Belongs to the Leg Lesser Yang (gallbladder) meridian.

INDICATIONS: Neckache, pain in legs, cramp of gastrocnemius.

12. KUANG-MING (GB 37)

LOCATION: 5 tsun above the lateral malleolus in front of the fibula.

ANATOMY: MUSCLE: Between long extensor of toes and short peroneal.
NERVE: Arising from L4–S1. Superficial layer: superficial peroneal. Deep layer: deep peroneal.

MERIDIAN: Belongs to the Leg Lesser Yang (gallbladder) meridian.

INDICATIONS: Myopia, asthenopia, night blindness, pain in the legs, hemicrania.

13. YANG-FU (GB 38)

LOCATION: 4 tsun above the lateral malleolus in front of the fibula.

ANATOMY: MUSCLE: Between long extensor of toes and short peroneal.
NERVE: Arising from L4–S1. Superficial layer: superficial peroneal. Deep layer: deep peroneal.

MERIDIAN: Belongs to the Leg Lesser Yang (gallbladder)

meridian.

INDICATIONS: Pain in all of the body, arthritis in knee, lumbago.

14. HSUAN-CHUNG (GB 39)

LOCATION: 3 tsun above the lateral malleolus in front of the fibula.

ANATOMY: MUSCLE: Between long extensor of toes and short peroneal.
NERVE: Arising from L4–S1. Superficial layer: superficial peroneal. Deep layer: deep peroneal.

MERIDIAN: Belongs to the Leg Lesser Yang (gallbladder) meridian, also is the joining point of the Leg Three Yang meridians.

INDICATIONS: Arthritis in the knees or ankles, hemiplegia.

15. CHIU-HSU (GB 40)

LOCATION: In the depression on the antero-inferior part of the lateral malleolus.

ANATOMY: MUSCLE: Origin of short extensor of toes.
NERVE: Arising from L4–S1. Superficial layer: dorsal cutaneous. Deep layer: deep peroneal.

MERIDIAN: An original point of the Leg Lesser Yang (gallbladder) meridian.

INDICATIONS: Lymphoglandulae subinguluales disturbance.

16. TSU-LIN-CHI (GB 41)

LOCATION: Between the 4th and 5th metatarsal bones 1.5 tsun behind Hsia-Hsi.

ANATOMY: NERVE: Arising from L4–S1. Lateral cutaneous of the dorsum of foot.

MERIDIAN: Belongs to the Leg Lesser Yang (gallbladder)

meridian. One connecting point goes through Tai-Mo.

INDICATIONS: Intercostal pain, lymphoglandulae cervicales, superficial disturbances, mastitis.

17. HSIA-HSI (GB 43)

LOCATION: ½ tsun behind the web between the 4th toe and little toe.

ANATOMY: NERVE: Arising from L5–S2. The dorsal nerve of the toes.

MERIDIAN: Belongs to the Leg Lesser Yang (gallbladder) meridian.

INDICATIONS: Deafness, dizziness, headache, intercostal pain.

18. YIN-MEN (B 51)

LOCATION: 6 tsun right above Wei-Chung (B 54) and in the center of the back of the thigh.

ANATOMY: MUSCLE: Semitendinosus.

NERVE: Superficial layer: dorsal femoral cutaneous arising from S1–S3. Deep layer: sciatic nerve arising from L4–S3.

MERIDIAN: Belongs to the Leg Greater Yang (bladder) meridian.

INDICATIONS: Pain in the lower limb, intervertebral disk, prolapse of lumbar, neck pain.

19. WEI-YANG (B 53)

LOCATION: On the lateral side of the popliteal fossa between the two tendons at the same level with Wei-Chung.

ANATOMY: MUSCLE: Medial tendon of the biceps femoris.

NERVE: Common peroneal from L2–L5, dorsal femoral cutaneous from S1–S3.

MERIDIAN: Belongs to the Leg Greater Yang (bladder)

meridian.

INDICATIONS: Gastrocnemius muscle cramp, lumbago, back pain.

20. WEI-CHUNG (B 54)

LOCATION: Midway of the popliteal fossa.

ANATOMY: MUSCLE: Between tendon of biceps femoris and tendon of semitendinosus.

NERVE: Superficial layer: dorsal femoral cutaneous from S1–S3. Deep layer: tibial nerve from L5–S2.

MERIDIAN: A join-point of the Leg Greater Yang (bladder) meridian.

INDICATIONS: Lumbago, backache, sciatica, hemiplegia, indigestion.

21. CHENG-SHAN (B 57)

LOCATION: Below the belly of the gastrocnemius muscle in the middle between the popliteal fossa and the heel.

ANATOMY: MUSCLE: The boundary between the belly and the tendon of gastrocnemius.

NERVE: Medial sural cutaneous and tibial nerve from S1–S2.

MERIDIAN: Belongs to the Leg Greater Yang (bladder) meridian.

INDICATIONS: Soreness and heaviness of the loins, back and legs, gastrocnemius muscle cramp, beri-beri, hemorrhoids, prolapse of anus.

22. FU-YANG (B 59)

LOCATION: 3 tsun postero-superior from the lateral malleolus opposite to Feng-Lung, behind Hsuan-Chung.

ANATOMY: MUSCLE: Short peroneal.

NERVE: Calf nerve from S1–S2.

MERIDIAN: Belongs to the Greater Yang (bladder) meridian.

INDICATIONS: Rheumatoid arthritis, nephritis, cystitis, eye disease, pain in the eyes.

23. KUN-LUN (B 60)

LOCATION: Between the lateral malleolus and the achilles tendon.

ANATOMY: MUSCLE: Short peroneal.
NERVE: Calf nerve from S1–S2.

MERIDIAN: Belongs to the Leg Greater Yang (bladder) meridian.

INDICATIONS: Headache, neckache, backache, lumbago, sciatica, palsy in lower limb, ankle pains.

24. CHING-KU (B 64)

LOCATION: On the lateral side of the foot, on the postero-inferior part of the tuberosity of the 5th metatarsal bone.

ANATOMY: MUSCLE: Below abductor of small toe.
NERVE: Superficial layer: lateral cutaneous of the dorsum of the foot. Deep layer: lateral plantar.

MERIDIAN: Belongs to Leg Greater Yang (bladder) meridian.

INDICATIONS: Headache, neckache, dizziness, epilepsy.

25. TAI-PAI (SP 3)

LOCATION: On the postero-inferior side of the distal end of the metatarsal bone of the big toe.

ANATOMY: MUSCLE: Abductor of great toe.
NERVE: Sciatic nerve from L3–L4. Branch of superficial peroneal from L4–S1.

MERIDIAN: Belongs to the Leg Greater Yin (spleen-pancreas) meridian.

INDICATIONS: Abdominal pain, diarrhea, constipation.

26. KUNG-SUN (SP 4)

LOCATION: 1 tsun behind the proximal end of the proximal phalange on the medial side of foot.

ANATOMY: MUSCLE: Abductor of great toe.
NERVE: Sciatic nerve from L3–L4. Branch of superficial peroneal from L4–S1.

MERIDIAN: Lo-Mo of the spleen meridian which separates into the stomach meridian, and passed by Chung-Mo.

INDICATIONS: Indigestion, abdominal pain, diarrhea, dysmenorrhea.

27. SAN-YIN-CHIAO (SP 6)

LOCATION: 3 tsun above the apex of the medial melleolus behind the tibia.

ANATOMY: MUSCLE: Anterior margin of soleus. In the deep layer is the long flexor of toes.
NERVE: Medial cutaneous branch of sciatic from L3–L4. In the deep layer is tibial nerve from L5–S2.

MERIDIAN: Belongs to the Leg Greater Yin (spleen) meridian and is the meeting point of the Leg Three Yin meridians.

INDICATIONS: Nocturnal pollution, impotence, premature ejaculation, nocturia, dysmenorrhea, irregular menstruation, neurasthenia, uterine hemorrhage, leukorrhagis, insomnia, hemiplegia, muscular atrophy of the lower limb, indigestion, diarrhea, hemorrhoids, intestinal colic, vaginodynia, diabetes.

28. YIN-LING-CHUAN (SP 9)

LOCATION: Under the knee joint on the medial border of the belly of the gastrocnemius.

ANATOMY: MUSCLE: Origin of soleus, gastrocnemius.
NERVE: Medial cutaneous branch of sciatic from L3–L4. In the deep layer is tibial nerve from L5–S2.

MERIDIAN: Belongs to the Leg Greater Yin (spleen) meridian

INDICATIONS: Abdominal distention, abdominal pain, ascites, ischuria, enuresia, retention of urine, nocturnal pollution, impotence, premature ejaculation, edema, pain in the lower limbs, loins and legs, dysentery, diseases of the gynecologic system.

29. HSUEH-HAI (SP 10)

LOCATION: 2 tsun above the medial border of the patella over the protuberance of the medial thigh, when the knee is bent.

ANATOMY: MUSCLE: Lower part of the medial great.
NERVE: Arising from L2–L4. Femoral and anterior femoral cutaneous.

MERIDIAN: Belongs to the Leg Greater Yin (spleen) meridian.

INDICATIONS: Irregular menstruation, metrorrhagia, urticaria, nettle rash.

30. YUNG-CHUAN (K 1)

LOCATION: ⅓ the distance from the center to the front of the plantar in the depression which is present when the foot is raised.

ANATOMY: MUSCLE: Aponeuroses plantaries. Tendon of short flexor of toes, long flexor of toes, in the deep layer is the interosseus.
NERVE: Common plantar of 2nd toe from L3–S1.

MERIDIAN: An original point of the kidney meridian.

INDICATIONS: Shock, epilepsy, hysteria, cerebral hemorrhage, infantile tetany.

31. CHAO-HAI (K 6)

LOCATION: In the depression directly below the medial malleolus.

ANATOMY: MUSCLE: Insertion of abductor of great toe.
Nerve: Medial cutaneous of leg from L5–S1.
In the deep layer is the tibial nerve from S1–S2.

MERIDIAN: Belongs to the Leg Lesser Yin (kidneys) meridian.

INDICATIONS: Neurasthenia, metromenorrohagia.

32. TAI-HSI (K 3)

LOCATION: Midway of the line connecting the border of the medial malleolus and the anterior border of the tendo calcaneus. On the same level with the tip of the medial malleolus.

ANATOMY: NERVE: Medial cutaneous of the leg from L5–S1. In the deep layer is the tibial nerve from S1–S2.

MERIDIAN: Belongs to Leg Lesser Yin (kidneys) meridian.

INDICATIONS: Nephritis, cysteria, palsy of lower limb.

33. TA-CHUNG (K 4)

LOCATION: ½ tsun behind Tai-Hsi between the achilles tendon and the calcaneus.

ANATOMY: MUSCLE: Achilles tendon.
NERVE: Medial cutaneous of the leg from L5–S1. In the deep layer is the medial calcaneus branch of the tibial nerve from S1–S2.

MERIDIAN: A Lo-Mo point of the kidneys meridian, separating into the bladder meridian.

INDICATIONS: Neurasthenia, asthma, constipation.

34. FU-LIU (K 7)

LOCATION: 2 tsun right below Tai-Hsi, in the front border of the achilles tendon.

ANATOMY: MUSCLE: Where the soleus communicates to the achilles tendon.
NERVE: Medial sural cutaneous from S1–S2. Medial cutaneous of the leg and tibial nerve.

MERIDIAN: Belongs to the Leg Lesser Yin (kidneys) meridian.

INDICATIONS: Nephritis, edema, night sweat, fever, testitis, lumbago.

35. HSING-CHIEN (LV 2)

LOCATION: In the web of the big toe and the second toe.

ANATOMY: NERVE: Where the dorsal plantar sends off the dorsal digital.

MERIDIAN: Belongs to the Leg Absolute Yin (liver) meridian.

INDICATIONS: Glaucoma, night sweat, intercostal pain, headache.

36. TAI-CHUNG (LV 3)

LOCATION: Between the 1st and the 2nd metatarsal bone, 1.5 tsun behind the web of the toe.

ANATOMY: MUSCLE: Lateral margin of long extensor of great toe.
NERVE: Branch of deep peroneal.

MERIDIAN: Belongs to the Leg Absolute Yin (liver) meridian.

INDICATIONS: High blood pressure, vertigo, diabetes, convulsion, laryngalgia, amenorrhea, inguinal colic, jaundice.

37. LI-KOU (LV 5)

LOCATION: 5 tsun above the medial malleolus on the posterior border of the tibia.

ANATOMY: NERVE: Anterior branch of sciatic from L3–L4.

MERIDIAN: Belongs to the Leg Absolute Yin (liver) meridian and passed by the gallbladder meridian.

INDICATIONS: Rupture, irregular menstruation, pain in the legs, urine hemorrhage.

38. CHUNG-TU (LV 6)

LOCATION: 7 tsun above the medial malleolus on the posterior border of the tibia.

ANATOMY: MUSCLE: Between tibia and soleus.
NERVE: Middle branch of sciatic.

MERIDIAN: Belongs to the Leg Absolute Yin (liver) meridian.

INDICATIONS: Rupture, arthritis in lower limb.

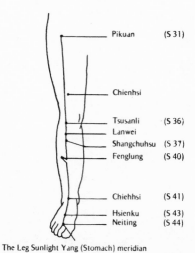

Pikuan	(S 31)
Chienhsi	
Tsusanli	(S 36)
Lanwei	
Shangchuhsu	(S 37)
Fenglung	(S 40)
Chiehhsi	(S 41)
Hsienku	(S 43)
Neiting	(S 44)

The Leg Sunlight Yang (Stomach) meridian

FIGURE 65. *Acupuncture points on the anterior surface of the lower limb.*

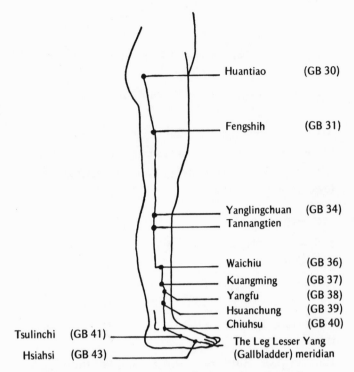

Huantiao	(GB 30)
Fengshih	(GB 31)
Yanglingchuan	(GB 34)
Tannangtien	
Waichiu	(GB 36)
Kuangming	(GB 37)
Yangfu	(GB 38)
Hsuanchung	(GB 39)
Chiuhsu	(GB 40)

Tsulinchi   (GB 41)

Hsiahsi   (GB 43)

The Leg Lesser Yang
(Gallbladder) meridian

FIGURE 66. *Acupuncture points on the lateral surface of the lower limb.*

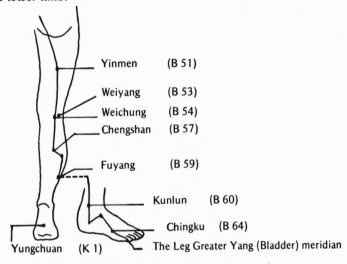

Yinmen	(B 51)
Weiyang	(B 53)
Weichung	(B 54)
Chengshan	(B 57)
Fuyang	(B 59)
Kunlun	(B 60)
Chingku	(B 64)

Yungchuan   (K 1)

The Leg Greater Yang (Bladder) meridian

FIGURE 67. *Acupuncture points on the posterior surface of the lower limb.*

162

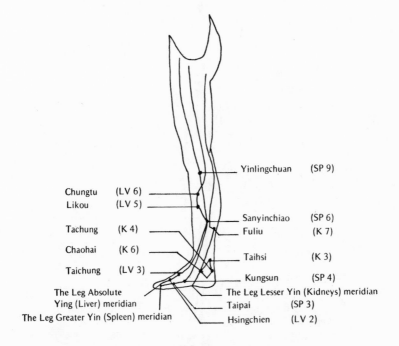

Chungtu   (LV 6)
Likou   (LV 5)

Tachung   (K 4)

Chaohai   (K 6)

Taichung   (LV 3)

The Leg Absolute
Ying (Liver) meridian

The Leg Greater Yin (Spleen) meridian

Yinlingchuan   (SP 9)

Sanyinchiao   (SP 6)
Fuliu   (K 7)

Taihsi   (K 3)

Kungsun   (SP 4)

The Leg Lesser Yin (Kidneys) meridian

Taipai   (SP 3)

Hsingchien   (LV 2)

FIGURE 68. *Acupuncture points on the medial surface of the lower limb.*

163

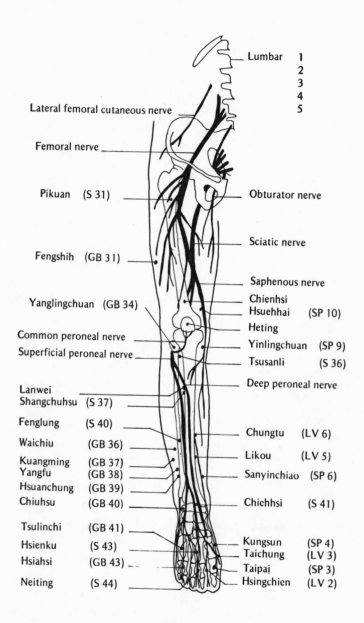

Lumbar 1
        2
        3
        4
        5

Lateral femoral cutaneous nerve

Femoral nerve

Pikuan   (S 31)

Obturator nerve

Sciatic nerve

Fengshih   (GB 31)

Saphenous nerve

Yanglingchuan (GB 34)

Chienhsi
Hsuehhai   (SP 10)

Common peroneal nerve

Heting

Superficial peroneal nerve

Yinlingchuan   (SP 9)

Tsusanli   (S 36)

Deep peroneal nerve

Lanwei
Shangchuhsu   (S 37)

Fenglung   (S 40)

Chungtu   (LV 6)

Waichiu   (GB 36)

Likou   (LV 5)

Kuangming   (GB 37)
Yangfu   (GB 38)

Sanyinchiao   (SP 6)

Hsuanchung   (GB 39)

Chiuhsu   (GB 40)

Chiehhsi   (S 41)

Tsulinchi   (GB 41)

Hsienku   (S 43)

Kungsun   (SP 4)

Taichung   (LV 3)

Hsiahsi   (GB 43)

Taipai   (SP 3)

Neiting   (S 44)

Hsingchien   (LV 2)

FIGURE 69. *Relation between acupuncture points on the anterior surface of the lower limb and the nerves.*
164

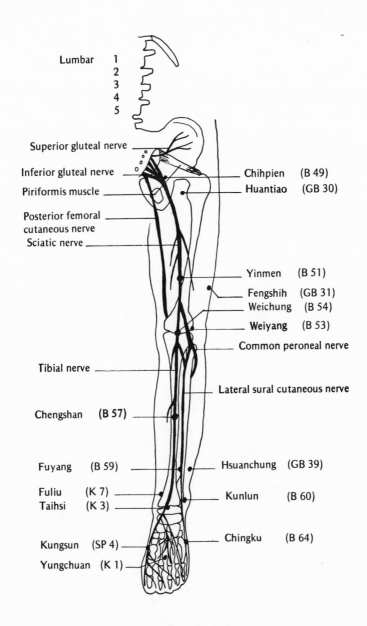

Lumbar 1
2
3
4
5

Superior gluteal nerve

Inferior gluteal nerve

Piriformis muscle

Posterior femoral cutaneous nerve

Sciatic nerve

Chihpien (B 49)
Huantiao (GB 30)

Yinmen (B 51)
Fengshih (GB 31)
Weichung (B 54)
Weiyang (B 53)
Common peroneal nerve

Tibial nerve

Lateral sural cutaneous nerve

Chengshan (B 57)

Fuyang (B 59)

Hsuanchung (GB 39)

Fuliu (K 7)
Taihsi (K 3)

Kunlun (B 60)

Kungsun (SP 4)

Chingku (B 64)

Yungchuan (K 1)

FIGURE 70. *Relation between acupuncture points on the posterior surface of the lower limb and the nerves.*

165

15

ACUPUNCTURE POINTS ON THE AURICLE

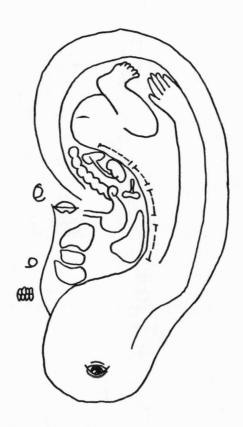

FIGURE 71. *Distribution order of ear points.*

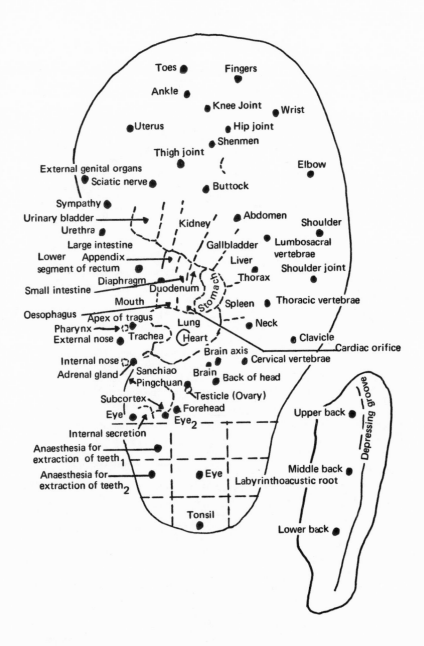

Toes
Fingers
Ankle
Knee Joint
Wrist
Uterus
Hip joint
Shenmen
Thigh joint
Elbow
External genital organs
Sciatic nerve
Buttock
Sympathy
Urinary bladder
Abdomen
Shoulder
Urethra
Kidney
Large intestine
Gallbladder
Lumbosacral
vertebrae
Lower Appendix
Liver
segment of rectum
Thorax
Shoulder joint
Diaphragm
Duodenum
Stomach
Small intestine
Mouth
Spleen
Thoracic vertebrae
Oesophagus
Apex of tragus
Lung
Neck
Pharynx
Trachea
Heart
External nose
Clavicle
Brain axis
Cardiac orifice
Internal nose
Cervical vertebrae
Adrenal gland
Sanchiao
Brain
Back of head
Pingchuan
Testicle (Ovary)
Subcortex
Forehead
Eye
Eye₂
Upper back
Internal secretion
Anaesthesia for
extraction of teeth₁
Anaesthesia for
Eye
Middle back
extraction of teeth₂
Labyrinthoacustic root
Tonsil
Lower back
Depressing groove

167

TABLE 13. *Locations of Acupuncture Points on the Auricle.*

	NAME OF POINTS	LOCATION
Crus of the Helix	Diaphragm	At the lower part of the crus of the helix.
Helix	Lower segment of the rectum	At the anterior portion of the helix with the same level of the acupuncture point of the large intestine.
	Urethra	At the anterior part of the helix with the same level of the acupuncture point of the urinary bladder.
	External genital organs	At the anterior part of the helix with the same level of the inferior crus of the antihelix.
Scapha	Fingers	At the scapha above the level of the auricular tubercle.
	Wrist	At the scapha with the same level of the auricular tubercle.
	Elbow	At the scapha lying between the acupuncture points of the wrist and elbow.
	Shoulder	At the scapha with the same level of the supratragic notch (incisura anterior).
	Shoulder joint	At the scapha lying between the acupuncture point of the shoulder and clavicle.
	Clavicle	At the scapha with the same level of the acupuncture point of the neck.
Superior Crus of the Antihelix	Toes	At the postero-superior part of superior crus of the antihelix.
	Ankle	At the antero-superior part of the superior crus of the antihelix.
Inferior Crus of the Antihelix	Sciatic nerve	At the middle point of superior border of the inferior crus of the antihelix (slightly towards the anterior side).
	Buttock	At the middle point of the superior border of the inferior crus of the antihelix (slightly towards the posterior side).
Antihelix	Knee Joint	At the superior crus of the antihelix, with the same level of the superior border of inferior crus of the antihelix.
	Abdomen	At the antihelix, with the same level of the lower border of the inferior crus of the antihelix.

168

TABLE 13. *Locations of Acupuncture Points on the Auricle. (Continued)*

	NAME OF POINTS	LOCATION
	Thorax	At the antihelix, with the same level of the supratragic incisure.
	Neck	At the notch between the border line of the antihelix and antitragus.
	Lumbo Sacral Vertebrae	A series of the acupuncture points of the vertebral column, lying along the curved brim of the cavum conchae on the antihelix. This line of the acupuncture points could be separated by the same level of the acupuncture
	Thoracic vertebrae	point of the lower segment of rectum and the same level of the acupuncture points of the shoulder joint into three segments. The upper segment belonging to the field of the lumbo-
	Cervical vertebrae	sacral vertebrae; the middle segment, the cervical vertebrae.
Triangular Fossa	Shen-Men	At the bifurcation of the crura of the antihelix.
	Uterus	At the middle point of the anterior portion of the triangular fossa just behind the anterior portion of the helix.
	Sympathy	At the border line between the brim of the inferior crus of the antihelix and curved brim of the anterior portion of the helix.
	Hip Joint	At the superior crus of the antihelix and the postero-inferior part of the acupuncture point of the knee joint.
Tragus	External Nose	At the central point of the root region of the tragus.
	Pharynx and Larynx	At the inner surface of the tragus opposite to the orifice of the external auditory meatus.
	Internal Nose	At the inner surface of the tragus, slightly below the acupuncture points of the pharynx and larynx.
	Apex of Tragus	The upper projection of the tragus (at the upper brim of the projection if only one projection is found).
	Adrenal Gland	The lower projection of the tragus (at the lower brim of the projection if only one projection is found).
Antitragus	Brain Axis	At the central point of the supra-tragic incisure.

169

	Brain point	On the lateral side of the antitragus, in the middle of the line connecting Brain Axis and Ping-Chuan.
	Ping-Chuan	At the apex of the antitragus (may locate at the central point of the brim of the antitragus if the apex of the antitragus is not prominent).
	Subcortex	At the inner surface of the antitragus.
	Testicle (Ovary)	About 0.2 mm. inside the acupuncture point of the parotid at the medial side of the antitragus.
	Back of Head	At the postero-superior part of the antitragus.
	Forehead	At the antero-interior part of the antitragus.
Intertragic Incisure	Eye 1, 2	At the inferior part of the intertragic incisure with the acupuncture point of the eye 1 in front and eye 2 behind.
Surroundings of the Crus of the Helix	Esophagus	At the upper portion of the cavum conchae just below the crus of the helix.
	Cardiac Orifice	At the upper portion of the cavum conchae and just below the crus of the helix. Its acupuncture point lies behind that of the esophagus.
	Stomach	At the upper portion of the cavum conchae and just below the disappearance of the crus of the helix.
	Duodenum	Lying above the crus of the helix opposite to the acupuncture point of the cardiac orifice.
	Small Intestine	At the lower portion of the cymba conchae and above the crus of the helix. It lies at point slightly lateral to one-half of the crus of the helix.
	Large Intestine	At the antero-interior portion of cymba conchae and just above the crus of the helix.
	Appendix	Just above the crus of the helix and lying among the acupuncture points of the large intestine and the small intestine.
Cymba Conchae	Urinary Bladder	At the antero-superior part of the cymba conchae, just below the inferior crus of the antihelix.
	Kidney	Lying in the upper part of the cymba conchae at the superior portion of the acupuncture point of the small intestine.

TABLE 13. *Locations of Acupuncture Points on the Auricle. (Continued)*

NAME OF POINTS		LOCATION
	Pancreas, Gallbladder	At the posterior part of the cymba conchae, just anterior to the acupuncture point of the thoracic vertebrae. This point lies between the acupuncture points of the liver and kidney. (On the left auricle, this point represents the pancreas, while on the right, the gallbladder.)
	Liver	Lying immediately posterior to the acupuncture point of the stomach in the postero-inferior part of the cymba conchae.
	Spleen	The lower half of the liver on the left auricle (on the right auricle the point of the liver remains exclusive.)
Cavum Conchae	Mouth	At the posterior wall of the orifice of the external auditory meatus.
	Heart	The acupuncture point lying at the center of the deepest position of the cavum conchae.
	Lung	Lying around the circumference of the acupuncture point of the heart.
	Trachea	Between mouth and heart.
	Internal Secretion	The bottom part of the intertragic incisure.
	San Chiao	The area between mouth, heart and internal secretion.
Auricular-lobe	Anaesthesia for extraction of teeth 1	At the postero-inferior part of the 1st area.
	Anaesthesia for extraction of teeth 2	At the central point of the 4th area.
	Eye	At the central point of the 5th area.
	Tonsils	At the central point of the 8th area.
Back of the Auricle	Depressing Groove	A curved vertical groove on the back of the auricle.
	Upper Back	At the upper cartilaginous eminence.
	Middle Back	Lying between the acupuncture points of the upper back and lower back.
	Lower Back	At the lower cartilaginous eminence.
	Labyrintho-acoustic root	On the border of the back of the auricle and the midpoint of mastoid process, on the ear-root on the level of the crus of the helix.

TABLE 14. *Ear-Needle Treatment for Reference.*

Subject	Diseases	Major Points	For Use
Internal	Infectious Diseases	Common Cold	Internal nose; adrenal gland; forehead; lung.	Subcortex; back of head.
		Varicella	Lung; internal secretion; adrenal gland; back of head; Shen-men.	
		Epidemic Parotitis	Parotid gland; internal secretion; cheeks.	
		Acute and Chronic Infectious Hepatitis	Liver; sympathy; Shen-men; spleen.	Kan-yang gallbladder; internal secretion; kidney.
		Pertussis	Lung; bronchi; adrenal gland; Shen-men; Ping-chuan.	Sympathy; back of head.
		Bacterial Dysentery	Large intestine; small intestine; lower segment of the rectum; Shen-men; internal secretion; back of head.	
		Phthisis	Lung; thorax; adrenal gland; internal secretion.	Subcortex; San-chiao.
		Malaria	Subcortex; internal secretion; liver; spleen.	
	Diseases of the Digestive System	Acute and Chronic Gastritis	Stomach; sympathy; Shen-men.	Spleen; abdomen.
		Gastric Ulcer	Stomach; sympathy; Shen-men.	Subcortex; duodenum.
		Duodenal Ulcer	Duodenum; sympathy; Shen-men.	Subcortex; stomach.

TABLE 14. *Ear-Needle Treatment for Reference. (Continued)*

SUBJECT		DISEASES	MAJOR POINTS	FOR USE
		Gastroptosis	Stomach; sympathy; subcortex.	Shen-men; liver.
		Spasm of the Stomach	Stomach; liver; sympathy; Shen-men.	Upper abdomen, lower abdomen.
		Gastro-enteric Neurosis	Stomach; liver; sympathy; Shen-men.	Duodenum.
		Musculophrenic Spasm	Diaphragm; Shen-men; subcortex.	
		Enteritis	Large intestine; lower segment of the rectum; sympathy; Shen-men.	Small intestine spleen.
Internal	Diseases of the Digestive System	Anaphylactic colitis.	Large intestine; internal secretion; sympathy.	Shen-men; small intestine.
		Intestinal Tuberculosis	Large intestine; small intestine; sympathy; Shen-men; internal secretion.	Back of head; San-chiao.
		Indigestion	Small intestine; stomach; pancreas-gallbladder; sympathy; spleen.	Large intestine; San-chiao; Shen-men.
		Nausea Vomiting	Stomach; Shen-men; back of head; sympathy.	Subcortex; esophagus.
		Diarrhea	Large intestine; small intestine; sympathy; Shen-men.	Lower segment of the rectum; spleen.
		Constipation	Large intestine; lower segment of the rectum; subcortex of the adrenal.	Sympathy.
		Distended Abdomen	Small intestine; large intestine; stomach; sympathy.	Abdomen; San-chiao.

173

	Intestinal Colic	Small intestine; sympathy; Shen-men.	Upper abdomen; lower abdomen.
	Functional Disturbance of the Stomach and Intestine	Stomach; small intestine; large intestine; sympathy.	Shen-men; spleen; San-chiao.
Diseases of the Respiratory System	Bronchitis	Bronchi; Shen-men; Ping-chuan; adrenal gland.	Sympathy; back of head.
	Lobar Pneumonia	Lung; thorax; adrenal gland; internal secretion.	Shen-men; subcortex.
	Broncho-pneumonia	Lung; bronchi; sympathy; Shen-men; Ping-chuan.	Adrenal gland; back of head; internal secretion.
	Asthma	Sympathy; Shen-men; Ping-chuan; adrenal gland.	Lung; back of head; internal secretion.
	Alveolar Emphysema	Lung; bronchi; sympathy; Shen-men; Ping-chuan.	Back of head; adrenal gland.
	Pleurisy	Lung; thorax; adrenal gland; internal secretion.	Subcortex; San-chiao.
	Pleural Adhesions	Thorax; adrenal gland; internal secretion.	Subcortex; Shen-men.
	Cough	Shen-men; Ping-chuan; adrenal gland.	Back of head; lung.
	Pressure on Chest	Sympathy; heart; thorax.	Back of head; lung.
	Chest Pain	Corresponds to the locality; Shen-men.	

Subject	Diseases	Major Points	For Use
Diseases of the Circulatory System	Myocarditis	Heart; small intestine; sympathy; Shen-men.	Back of head.
	Rheumatoid Cardiopathy	Heart; internal secretion; sympathy; Shen-men.	Small intestine; subcortex.
	Cardiac Arrhythmia	Heart; sympathy; Shen-men.	Subcortex.
	High Blood Pressure	Depressing point; sympathy; Shen-men; heart.	Depressing groove (blood letting).
	Low Blood Pressure	Sympathy; heart; back of head; adrenal gland.	
	Buerger's Disease	Sympathy; kidney; heart; adrenal gland; liver; spleen.	Internal secretion; subcortex; back of head.
	Inflamation in Pulse Artery	Sympathy; kidney; heart; adrenal gland; liver.	Spleen; back of head; internal secretion.
	Peripheral Circulatory Disturbances	Corresponds to the locality; internal secretion; adrenal gland.	
Diseases of the Blood System	Hypoferric Anemia	Liver; spleen; internal secretion; diaphragm.	Stomach; small intestine.
	Leukopenia	Liver; spleen; heart; kidney; internal secretion.	Back of head; diaphragm; sympathy.

	Thrombopenic Purpura	Liver; spleen; diaphragm; sympathy; Shen-men; internal secretion.	Back of head; heart.
Diseases of the Urinary and Generative System	Acute Nephritis	Kidney; urinry bladder; sympathy; Shen-men; liver.	Adrenal gland; internal secretion.
	Nephropathic Syndrome	Kidney; urinary bladder; sympathy; Shen-men; ascites.	Adrenal gland.
	Pyelonephritis	Kidney; urinary bladder; sympathy; Shen-men; liver.	Adrenal gland; internal secretion.
	Failure of the Kidney Function	Kidney; urinary bladder; sympathy; Shen-men.	Adrenal gland; back of head.
	Hematuria	Kidney; urinary bladder; liver; diaphragm; adrenal gland.	
	Pollakisuria; Precipitant Urination	Urinary bladder; kidney; Shen-men.	Urethra; external genita organs.
	Retention of Urine	Kidney; urinary bladder; sympathy; external genital organs.	
	Incontinence of Urine	Urinary bladder; brain; point of support.	Subcortex.
	Impotence	Uterus; external genital organs; testicle; internal secretion; kidney.	Back of head; kidney.
	Ejaculatio praecox	Uterus; external genital organs; testicle; internal secretion; Shen-men.	

Subject	Diseases	Major Points	For Use
	Orchitis	Testicle; internal secretion; Shen-men; adrenal gland.	External genital organs.
	Epididymitis	Testicle; internal secretion; Shen-men; adrenal gland.	External genital organs; Ku-Kuan.
	Prostatitis	Prostate; urinary bladder; internal secretion; kidney.	Back of head.
Diseases of the Endocrine System	Hypophysial Dwarfism	Kidney; internal secretion; brain.	Testicle (male); ovary (female).
	Hypothyroidism	Thyroid; internal secretion; brain; Shen-men.	
	Hyperthyroidism	Thyroid; internal secretion; brain; Shen-men.	Cervical vertebrae.
	Sheehan's Disease	Brain; liver; spleen; sympathy; uterus; internal secretion.	
	Diabetes Insipidus	Brain; internal secretion; sympathy; Shen-men; kidney; urinary bladder.	
	Secretory Disturbances	Internal secretion, brain; subcortex; spleen.	Testicle (male); ovary (female).
	Gynecomastia	Internal secretion; brain; mammary gland.	
Diseases of the Locomotor System	Neck Pain	Internal secretion; brain; cervical vertebrae; neck; Shen-men.	
	Hypertrophic Spondylopathy	Corresponds to the locality; internal secretion; adrenal gland; subcortex.	Kidney; Shen-men.

	Periarthritis of the Shoulder	Shoulder joint; shoulder; Shen-men.	Clavicle; adrenal gland.
	Rheumatoid Arthritis	Shen-men; kidney; internal secretion; back of the head; corresponds to the locality.	Subcortex.
	Joint Friction	Corresponds to the locality; internal secretion; adrenal gland; subcortex.	Kidney; Shen-men
	Osteomalacia of the Patella	Corresponds to the locality; internal secretion; adrenal gland; subcortex.	Kidney; Shen-men.
Diseases of the Mental and Nervous System	Trigeminal Neuralgia	Cheeks; upper jaw; lower jaw; Shen-men; back of head.	External ear.
	Facial nerve Paralysis	Cheeks; back of head; eye; mouth.	Upper jaw; lower jaw; liver.
	Facial Spasms	Cheeks; Shen-men; subcortex; the sun.	
	Meniere's Disease	Kidney; Shen-men; back of head; internal ear.	Subcortex; stomach.
	Intercosta Neuralgia	Thorax; back of head.	
	Ischialgia	Ischium; Shen-men; kidney; back of head.	Adrenal gland.
	Multiple Neuritis	Corresponds to the locality; Shen-men; adrenal gland; internal secretion.	
	Amyotrophic lateral Sclerosis	Kidney; internal secretion; brain axis; back of head; San-chiao.	

Subject	Diseases	Major Points	For Use
	Cerebellar Ataxia	Brain axis; back of head; cervical vertebrae.	Kidney; Shen-men.
	Epilepsy	Shen-men; kidney; back of head; heart; stomach.	Subcortex.
	After-effects of Commotio Cerebri	Kidney; brain axis; back of head; Shen-men; heart.	Stomach; subcortex.
	After-effects of Cerebral Meningitis	Kidney; brain axis; back of head; Shen-men; heart.	Stomach; subcortex.
	After-effects of Infantile Paralysis	Corresponds to the locality; Shen-men; adrenal gland; internal secretion.	Subcortex; back of head.
Internal	After-effects of Cerebral Hemorrhage	Corresponds to the locality; Shen-men; adrenal gland; internal secretion.	Subcortex; back of head.
Diseases of the Mental and Nervous System	Atelencephalia	Kidney; back of the head; brain stem axis; Shen-men; subcortex.	Internal secretion; forehead.
	Migraine	The sun; Shen-men; kidney; subcortex.	
	Hyperhidrosis	Sympathy; lung; internal secretion; back of head; adrenal gland.	
	Headache; Dizziness	Back of head; forehead; Shen-men; subcortex.	

	Insomnia; Frequent Dreams	Shen-men; kidney; heart; back of head.	
	Neurasthenia	Heart; kidney; Shen-men; back of head; stomach.	Subcortex.
	Hysteria	Heart; kidney; Shen-men; brain axis; back of head; stomach.	Subcortex.
	Hysteric Paralysis	Subcortex; Shen-men; back of head; heart; corresponds to the locality.	Stomach; kidney.
	Hysteric Aphasia	Brain; back of head; heart; Shen-men; kidney; subcortex.	
	Schizophrenia	Kidney; Shen-men; back of head; heart; stomach; brain axis.	Subcortex.
	Hallucination	Kidney; liver; eye; back of head.	
Surgery	Furuncle, Carbuncle and Paronychia	Corresponds to the locality; Shen-men; back of head; adrenal gland.	
	Cellulitis	Corresponds to the locality; adrenal gland; Shen-men.	
	Erysipelas	Corresponds to the locality (momentary insertion); lung; back of head; adrenal gland; internal secretion; Shen-men.	
	Mastitis	Mammary gland; internal secretion; back of head; adrenal gland.	
	Mammary Abscess	Mammary gland; internal secretion; back of head; adrenal gland.	

180

Subject	Diseases	Major Points	For Use
Surgery	Acute and Chronic Appendicitis	Appendix; large intestine; sympathy; Shen-men.	
	Cholelithiasis	Gallbladder; sympathy; Shen-men.	Liver; duodenum.
	Round-Worms in the Biliary Tract.	Gallbladder; sympathy; Shen-men.	Liver; duodenum.
	Chronic Cholecystitis	Gallbladder; liver; sympathy; Shen-men.	
	Chronic Pancreatitis	Pancreas; internal secretion; sympathy; Shen-men.	Internal secretion
	Paralytic Intestinal Obstruction	Large intestine; small intestine; sympathy; subcortex; abdomen.	
	Renal Calculus	Kidney; ureter; sympathy; Shen-men.	
	Ureteral Calculus	Ureter; kidney; sympathy; Shen-men.	Subcortex
	Incomplete Hernia	Lower abdomen; subcortex; internal secretion.	
	Anal Fissure	Lower segment of the rectum; Shen-men.	Large intestine; spleen.
	Prolapse of Anus	Lower segment of the rectum; large intestine; subcortex.	Spleen
	Internal Piles; External Piles	Lower segment of the rectum; large intestine.	Subcortex; spleen; adrenal gland.

Cystitis	Urinary bladder; kidney; sympathy; Shen-men.	Back of head; adrenal gland.
Prostatitis	Prostate; urinary bladder; internal secretion; kidney.	Back of head.
Orchitis; Epididymitis	Testicle; internal secretion; Shen-men; adrenal gland.	External genital organs; Ku-kuan.
Fracture, Contusion, Sprain	Corresponds to the locality; Shen-men; kidney; subcortex.	Adrenal gland.
Habitual Dislocation of Joint.	Corresponds to the locality; internal secretion; adrenal gland; subcortex.	
Bone Spicule after Arthritis or Periostitis	Kidney; internal secretion; back of head; adrenal gland; corresponds to the locality.	
Dysmenorrhea	Uterus; internal secretion; sympathy; Shen-men.	
Amenorrhea	Uterus; internal secretion; ovary; adrenal gland; kidney.	
Functional Hemorrhage from the Uterus	Uterus; brain; internal secretion; liver; spleen; kidney.	Adrenal gland.
Leukorrhagia	Uterus; ovary; internal secretion.	
Endometritis	Uterus; ovary; internal secretion; adrenal gland.	External genital organs.

Gynecology

Subject	Diseases	Major Points	For Use
	Prolapse of the Uterus	Uterus; subcortex.	External genital organs.
	Chronic Pelviope—ritonitis	Uterus; ovary; internal secretion; pelvic cavity.	
	Adnexitis	Ovary; internal secretion; Shen-men.	Adrenal gland.
	Postnatal Involution Pain	Uterus; sympathy; Shen-men.	Subcortex
	Vulvar Pruritus	External genital organs (momentary insertion); back of head; adrenal gland; Shen-men; lung; internal secretion.	
Opthalmology	Hordeolum; Chalazion	Eye; liver; spleen.	
	Acute Conjunctivitis	Eye; liver.	
	Anaphylactic Conjuctivitis	Eye; liver; back of head; internal secretion.	
	Follicular Conjunctivitis	Eye; liver.	
	Electric Ophthalmitis	Kidney; liver; eye.	Shen-men
	Glaucoma	Kidney; liver; eye[1]; eye[2]; eye.	
	Papillitis	Kidney; liver; eye[1]; eye[2]; eye.	

Optic Atrophy	Kidney; liver; eye.	
Night Blindness	Liver; eye²; eye.	
Myopia	Kidney; liver; eye ^{2}; eye.	
Diffused light	Kidney; liver; eye; eye ^{2}; back of head.	
Diplopia	Kidney; liver; eye ^{2}; eye.	

Otorhinolaryngology

Tinnitus Aurium	Kidney; back of head; internal ear; external ear.	
Impaired Hearing	Kidney; back of head; internal ear; external ear.	
Furunculosis of the External Meatus	Kidney; internal ear; internal secretion.	External ear.
Otitis Media	Kidney; internal ear; internal secretion.	External ear.
Simple Rhinitis	Internal nose; adrenal gland; forehead.	Lung
Atrophic Rhinitis	Internal nose; adrenal gland; forehead.	
Anaphylactic Rhinitis	Internal nose; adrenal gland; forehead; internal secretion.	
Epistaxis	Internal nose; adrenal gland; forehead.	
Ulcerous Vestibulum Nasi	Internal nose; adrenal gland; forehead; lung.	
Nasosinulitis	Internal nose; adrenal gland; forehead.	

Subject	Diseases	Major Points	For Use
	Chronic Pharyngitis	Pharynx and larynx; Shen-men; heart; internal secretion.	Lung; Hou-ya
	Chronic Laryngitis	Pharynx and larynx; Shen-men; heart; internal secretion.	Internal secretion.
	Hoarseness	Pharynx and larynx; heart; lung; Shen-men.	
	Acute Tonsillitis	Tonsils; pharynx and larynx.	Hilix 1–hilix 6.
	Uvular Edema	Pharynx and larynx; Shen-men; adrenal gland.	
Stomatology	Decayed Teeth; Toothache	Shang-he (maxilla); Hsia-he (mandible); Shen-men; toothache.	Hou-ya
	Periodontitis	Shang-he (maxilla); Hsia-he (mandible); mouth; adrenal gland.	Kidney
	Retardation of the Development of Teeth	Shang-he (maxilla); Hsia-he (mandible); Shen-men; toothache.	Hou-ya
	Agomphiasis	Kidney; Shang-he (maxilla); Hsia-he (mandible); back of head.	
	Stomatocace	Mouth; internal secretion; Shen-men; tongue.	
Stomatology	Mycotic Stomatitis	Mouth; internal secretion; adrenal gland; spleen; back of head.	
	Glossitis	Tongue; internal secretion; heart.	

185

Dermatology	Folliculitis; Herpes Zoster	Corresponds to the locality (momentary insertion); lung; back of head; internal secretion; adrenal gland.
	Verruca Vulgaris	Lung; internal secretion; back of head; adrenal gland; corresponds to the locality (momentary insertion).
	Pernio (1–2 degrees)	Corresponds to the locality; Shen-men; back of head; spleen; adrenal gland.
	Dermatitis Solaris	Shen-men; lung; internal secretion; adrenal gland.
	Eczema; Verrucaplana	Lung; secretion; back of head; large intestine.
	Infantile Eczema	Corresponds to the locality; lung; back of head; internal secretion.
	Anaphylactic Dermatitis	Lung; internal secretion; back of head; adrenal gland; corresponds to the locality (momentary insertion).
	Urticaria	Lung; Shen-men; back of head; internal secretion; adrenal gland.
	Cutaneous Pruritus	Shen-men; lung; back of head; internal secretion; adrenal gland.
	Neurodermatitis	Corresponds to the locality (momentary insertion); back of head; internal secretion; adrenal gland.
	Chorionitis	Lung; back of head; internal secretion; adrenal gland; liver; spleen; brain.

Dermatitis Seborrhoica	Lung; internal secretion; spleen; back of head; adrenal gland.
Vitiligo	Lung; internal secretion; back of head; adrenal gland; corresponds to the locality (momentary insertion).
Alopecia	Kidney; lung; internal secretion; back of head.
Alopecia Areata	Corresponds to the locality (momentary insertion); kidney; lung; internal secretion.
Acne	Lung; internal secretion; testicle; cheeks (momentary insertion).
Dermatology Rosacea	External nose (momentary insertion); lung; internal secretion; adrenal gland.
Miliaria	Lung; internal secretion; adrenal gland; back of head; Shen-men.
The Others Heat Stroke	Back of head; heart; subcortex; adrenal gland. Brain
Shock	Adrenal gland; back of head; heart.
Drunkenness	Back of head; forehead; subcortex.
Seasickness; Trainsickness	Back of head; stomach. Internal ear; Shen-men.
Edema of Indistinct Origin	Kidney; urinary bladder; heart; liver; sympathy; internal secretion.
Low Grade Fever of Indistinct Origin	Apex of the auricle; apex of tragus; adrenal gland (blood letting); internal secretion; liver; spleen; Shen-men.
Multiple Lymphnodoncus	Ku-kuan; back of head; internal secretion.

PART III

Treatment for the Common Diseases

FOREWORD

Part III lists several prescriptions for specific diseases. The publication of these prescriptions, many of which up to now have been "secret," serves a twofold purpose. First, they may be used as examples of the various factors that must be considered by those who are learning to formulate their own prescriptions. Second, they can be applied using the mediums of acupressure, massage, or if qualified—needling. It should always be remembered that Chinese medicine is preventive; if these prescriptions are applied to one's own body or to that of another, they will balance the energy and those "indications" of disease will never develop.

16

INTERNAL DISEASES

1. COMMON COLD

PRESCRIPTION:

BODY POINTS: Feng-Chih (GB 20), Ho-Ku (LI 4), Fu-Liu (K 7).

For *fever,* add Ta-Chui (TU 14).

For *headache,* add Chu-Chih (LI 11).

For *nasal congestion,* add Ying-Hsiang (LI 20).

For *coughing,* add Chih-Tse (L 5).

For *phlegm,* add Fu-Tu (LI 18), Fung-Lung (S 40).

EAR POINTS: Inner nose, subcortex.

METHOD OF TREATMENT: Mostly using *dispersion;* using *stimulation* for assistance only. One treatment daily, continuing as needed.

ACUPRESSING:

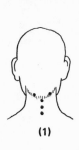
(1)

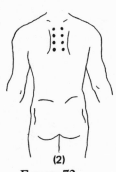
(2)

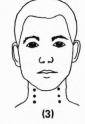
(3)

FIGURE 72.

PREVENTION: Tsu-San-Li (S 36)—Needling. One treatment daily, continuing for three days.

2. HEPATITIS

PRESCRIPTION:

BODY POINTS: Kan-Shu (B 18), Tan-Shu (B 19), Tsu-San-Li (S 36), Tai-Chung (K 3).
For *pain*, add Chu-Hsu (GB 40).
For *dropsy*, add San-Yin-Chiao (SP 6), Kuan-Yuan (JEN 4).
For *fever*, add Ta-Chui (TU 14).
For *jaundice*, add Yang-Ling-Chuan (GB 34), Chih-Yang (TU 9).

EAR POINTS: Liver, sympathetic, Shen-Men, internal secretion, gallbladder.

METHOD OF TREATMENT: Dispersion—Must be very strong action. Acute: One treatment daily, continuing as needed. Chronic: One treatment every three or four days with seven treatments making *one period of treatment*. The treatments may be continued for three to four periods.

ACUPRESSING: For assistance only.

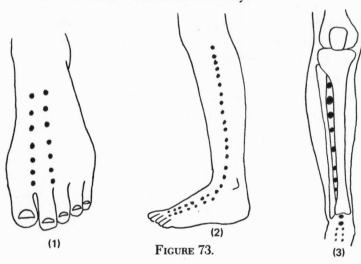

(1)　　　(2)　　　(3)

FIGURE 73.

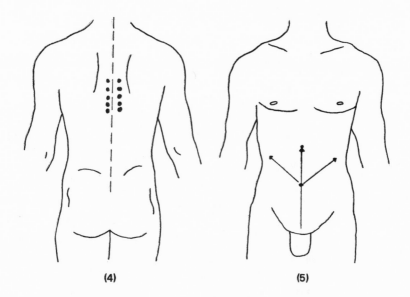

(4)   (5)

3. BRONCHITIS

PRESCRIPTION:

BODY POINTS: Tien-Tu (JEN 22), Fei-Shu (B 13), Chih-Tse (L 5).
For *phlegm,* add Feng-Lung (S 40).
For *fever,* add Ta-Chui (TU 14), Ho-Ku (LI 4).
Chronic: must associate Tien-Tu (JEN 22) and Feng-Lung (S 40).

EAR POINTS: Lung, bronchi, adrenal gland, Shen-Men.

METHOD OF TREATMENT: Stimulation—One treatment daily, continuing as needed.

PREVENTION: Fei-Shu (B 13), Ta-Chui (TU 14), Kuan-Yuan (JEN 4), Tsu-San-Li (S 36). One treatment daily, twelve treatments making *one period of treatment,* after which there should be *three days of rest.* The treatments may be continued for up to three to five periods.

ACUPRESSING:

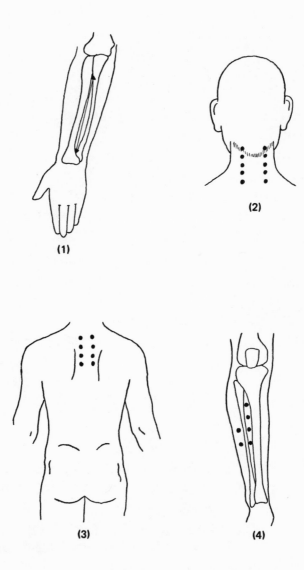

FIGURE 74.

4. ASTHMA

PRESCRIPTION:

BODY POINTS: 1. Paroxysmal: Tien-Yu (JEN 22), Nei-Kuan (HC 6), Fei-Shu (B 13), Shan-Chung (JEN 17).
For *phlegm,* add Kun-Tsui (L 6), Feng-Lung (S 40).
2. Remissional: Ta-chui (TU 14), Fei-Shu (B 13), Tsu-San-Li (S 36).
For *kidney*-Hsü, add Shen-Shu (B 23), Kuan-Yuan (JEN 4).
For *spleen*-Hsü, add Pi-Shu (B 30), Chung-Wan (JEN 12)

EAR POINTS: Lung, bronchi, trachae, Shen-Men, adrenal gland, internal secretion. Two to three points may be selected for use in each treatment.

METHOD OF TREATMENT: 1. Paroxysmal: *Dispersion* once daily. 2. Remissional: *Stimulation* once every two days.

ACUPRESSING: The same as No. 3.

5. PALPITATION (VALVULAR DISEASE OF THE HEART)

PRESCRIPTION:

BODY POINTS: Feng-Chih (GB 20), Ta-chui (TU 14), Hsin-Shu (B 15), Chung-Wan (JEN 12).
For *edema,* add Shen-Shu (B 23), Tsu-San-Li (S 36), San-Yin-Chiao (SP 6).

EAR POINTS: Heart, small intestine, sympathetic, Shen-Men.

METHOD OF TREATMENT: *Dispersion* and *Stimulation* One treatment daily, continuing as needed.

ACUPRESSING:

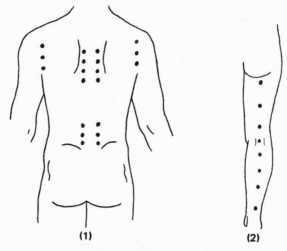

(1) (2)

FIGURE 75.

6. PNEUMONIA

PRESCRIPTION:

BODY POINTS: Fei-Shu (B 13), Ta-Chui (TU 14) Chu-Chih (LI 11), Nei-Kuan (P 6), Wai-Kuan (TH 6).

For *headache or fever,* add Feng-Chih (GB 20), Ho-Ku (LI 4), Fu-Liu (K 7), Shou-Chung (H 9).

For *coughing or pain in the chest,* add Chih-Tse (L 5), Tai-Yuen (L 9), Chung-Wan (JEN 12).

EAR POINTS: Lung, chest, adrenal gland, bronchi.

METHOD OF TREATMENT: One treatment daily, continuing as needed.

ACUPRESSING: For assistance only.

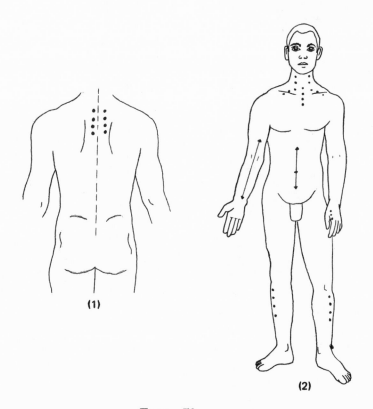

(1)

(2)

FIGURE 76.

7. CARDIAC COLIC

PRESCRIPTION:

BODY POINTS: Nei-kuan (HC 6), Hsin-Shu (B 15), Chien-Cheng (SI 9), Chieng-Ching (GB 21), Tau-San-Li (S 36).

EAR POINTS: Heart, small intestine, sympathetic, internal secretion.

METHOD OF TREATMENT: One treatment daily or every three days, continuing as needed. Both *Dispersion* and *Stimulation.*

ACUPRESSING:

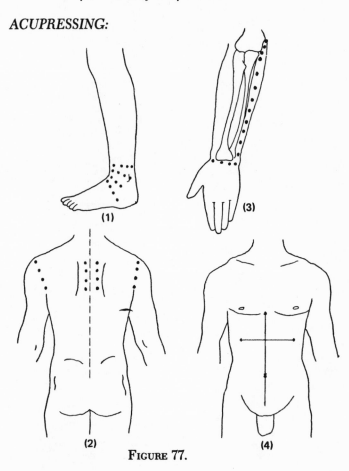

(1)

(2)

(3)

(4)

FIGURE 77.

8. CARDIAC ARRHYTHMIA

PRESCRIPTION:

BODY POINTS: Nei-Kuan (HC 6), Shang-Chung (JEN 17), Hsin-Shu (B 15), Feng-Chih (GB 20).

EAR POINTS: Heart, kidney, internal secretion, Shen-Men, small intestine.

METHOD OF TREATMENT: Stimulation—One treatment daily or every three days, continuing as needed.

ACUPRESSING: The same as No. 7.

9. TUBERCULOSIS—IN LUNGS

PRESCRIPTION:

BODY POINTS: Fei-Shu (B 13), Feng-Lung (S 40), Chih-Tse (L 5), Tsu-San-Li (S 36).

For *phlegm,* add Feng-Men (B 12), Tai-Yuan (L 9).

For *hemoptysis,* add Kun-Chui (L 6), Ke-Shu (B 17), San-Yin-Chiao (SP 6).

For *fever,* add Ta-Chui (TU 14), Chieng-Shih (HC 5).

For *sweat,* add Hou-Hsi (SI 3), Fu-Liu (K 7).

For *lack of appetite,* add Chung-Wan (JEN 12), Pi-Shu (B 20).

EAR POINTS: Lung, bronchi, trachae, sympathetic, adrenal gland. (For assistance only.)

ACUPRESSING: For assistance only.

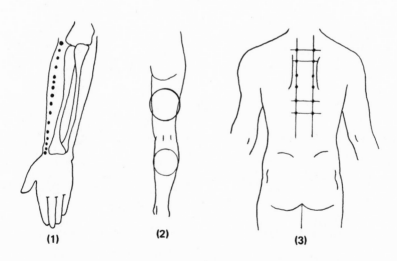

(1)   (2)   (3)

FIGURE 78.

10. HIGH BLOOD PRESSURE

PRESCRIPTION:

BODY POINTS: Chu-Chih (LI 11), Tsu-San-Li (S 36).
For *vertigo* or *headache,* add Feng-Chih (GB 20), Tai-Chung (LV 3), Jen-Ying (S 9).

EAR POINTS: Hypertension point, depressing point, sympathetic, Shen-Men, heart.

METHOD OF TREATMENT: Using *Stimulation* mostly, leave the needles in for more than 30 minutes. One treatment daily, continuing as needed.

ACUPRESSING:

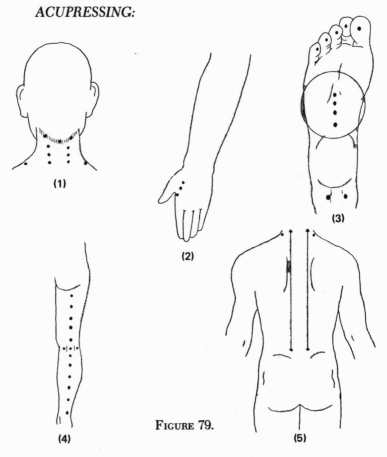

(1)

(2)

(3)

(4)

(5)

FIGURE 79.

11. LOW BLOOD PRESSURE

PRESCRIPTION:

BODY POINTS: Su-Liao (TU 25), Nei-Kuan (HC 6), Tai-Chung (LV 3).

EAR POINTS: Sympathetic, Shen-Men, heart, adrenal gland.

METHOD OF TREATMENT: Stimulation.—One treatment daily, continuing as needed.

ACUPRESSING:

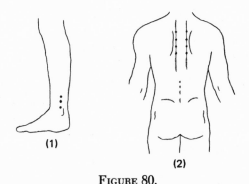

(1)

(2)

FIGURE 80.

12. CHRONIC GASTRIC ULCER

PRESCRIPTION:

BODY POINTS: Chung-Wan (JEN 12), Nei-Kuan (HC 6), Tsu-San-Li (S 36), Wei-Shu (B 21).

For *indistinct pain,* add Yang-Ling-Chuen (GB 34).

For *abdominal distention,* add Tien-Shu (S 25).

For *colic,* add Wai-Kuan (TH 5).

For *blood in stool,* add Tai-Chung (LV 3).

For *high gastric acidity,* add Tsu-San-Li (S 36), if *low,* use Shou-San-Li (LI 10), Shang-Wan (JEN 13).

EAR POINTS: Sympathetic, Shen-Men, stomach, subcortex, duodenum.

METHOD OF TREATMENT: Using *Stimulation*, leaving needles in 30 minutes or more. One treatment daily or every three days, continuing as needed.

ACUPRESSING:

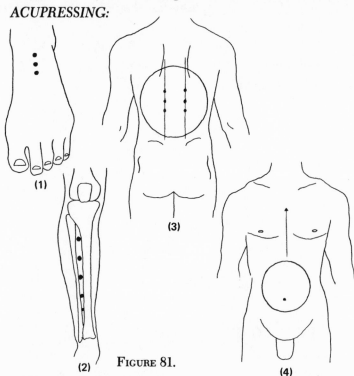

(1)

(2)   FIGURE 81.

(3)

(4)

13. CHRONIC DIARRHEA

PRESCRIPTION:

BODY POINTS: Tien-Shu (S 25), Chi-Hai (JEN 6), Kuan-Yuen (JEN 4), Ta-Hun (SP 15).
For *indigestion,* add Chung-Wan (JEN 12).
For *water,* add Pi-Shu (B 20).
For *weakness,* add Shen-Shu (B 23), Tai-Hsi (K 3).

EAR POINTS: Small and large intestine, sympathetic, Shen-Men.

METHOD OF TREATMENT: Using *Stimulation*, one treatment daily, seven treatments making *one period of treatment*. Treatments may be continued up to three periods.

ACUPRESSING:

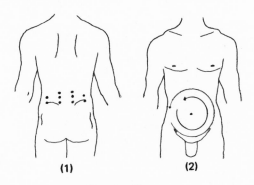

(1)   (2)

FIGURE 82.

14. GASTRO-ENTERITIS

PRESCRIPTION:

BODY POINTS: Chung-Wan (JEN 12), Tien-Shu (S 25), Nei-Kuan (HC 6), Tsu-San-Li (S 36).
For *fever*, add Chu-Chih (LI 11), Ta-Chui (TU 14).
For *vomiting*, add Ho-Ku (LI 4), Yung-Chuan (K 1).
For *straining*, add Yang-Ling-Chuan (GB 34), Wei-Chung (B 54).

EAR POINTS: Sympathetic, stomach, small and large intestine.

METHOD OF TREATMENT: Using *Dispersion first*, then *Stimulation*, leave needles in for more than 30 minutes. One or two treatments daily, continuing as needed.

ACUPRESSING: For assistance only.

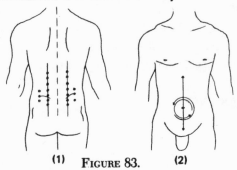

(1)   FIGURE 83.   (2)

15. INTESTINAL TROUBLE

PRESCRIPTION:

BODY POINTS: 1. *Intestinal obstruction* (paralyzing): Tien-Shu (S 25), Chi-Hai (JEN 6), Ta-Chang-Shu (B 25).
2. *Intestinal spasm:* Nei-Kuan (HC 6), Chung-Wan (JEN 12), Tien-Shu (S 25).

EAR POINTS: Small and large intestine, sympathetic, internal secretion.

METHOD OF TREATMENT: One treatment every two days, with seven treatment making *one period of treatment.* The treatments may be continued up to three or four periods. Four to seven days of rest should be taken between each two periods of treatment. Using *Stimulation,* leave needles in for more than 30 minutes.

ACUPRESSING:

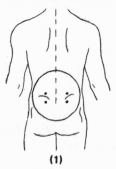
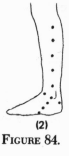
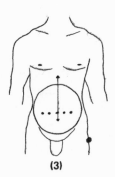

(2)
FIGURE 84.

(1)   (3)

16. CONSTIPATION

PRESCRIPTION:

BODY POINTS: Wei-Shu (B 21), Ta-Chang-Shu (B 25), Chi-Hai (JEN 6), Tien-Shu (S 25), Chang-Chiang (TU 1), Yang-Ling-Chuan (GB 34).

EAR POINTS: Lower segment of the rectum, large intestine, subcortex.

METHOD OF TREATMENT: 1. Shih—*Dispersion.* 2. Hsü—*Stimulation.* One treatment daily, continuing as needed.

ACUPRESSING:

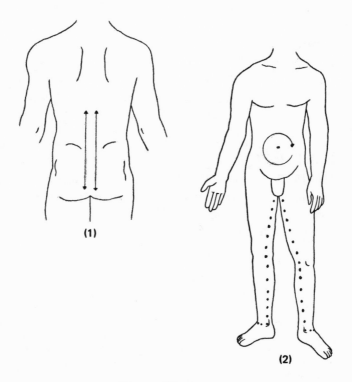

(1)

(2)

FIGURE 85.

17. APPENDICITIS

PRESCRIPTION:

BODY POINTS: Tien-Shu (S 25), Shang-Chu-Sheh (S 37), Lan-Wei-Tien (new point—1 tsun above Shang-Chu-Sheh-S 37).
For *fever,* add Chu-Chih (LI 11) and Ta-Chui (TU 14).
For *vomiting,* add Chung-Wan (JEN 12).

EAR POINTS: Vermiform appendix, sympathetic, large intestine, Shen-Men.

METHOD OF TREATMENT: Using *Dispersion,* one treatment or several treatments daily, continuing as needed.

ACUPRESSING: Forbidden

18. HEAD-ACHE

PRESCRIPTION:

BODY POINTS: Ho-Ku (LI 4), Wai-Kuan (TH 5), Feng-Chih (GB 20), Pai-Hui (TU 20), Yin-Tang (strange point—the center of the eyebrows), Kun-Lun (B 60), Yung-Chuan (K 1).

EAR POINTS: Subcortex, forehead, Shen-men, occiput.

METHOD OF TREATMENT: 1. Acute: *Dispersion.* 2. Chronic: *Stimulation.* One treatment daily for a week, continuing as needed.

ACUPRESSING:

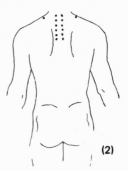

(1) FIGURE 86. (2)

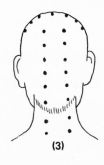

(3)

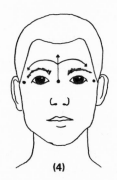

(4)

19. DIZZINESS

PRESCRIPTION:

BODY POINTS: Nei-Kuan (HC 6), Tai-Chung (LV 3), Er-Men (TH 21), I-Feng (TH 17), Chi-Hai (JEN 6), Chung-Wan (JEN 12), Feng-Lung (S 40).

EAR POINTS: Kidney, Shen-Men, back of head (occiput), stomach.

METHOD OF TREATMENT: Using *Stimulation*, one treatment daily for a week, continuing as needed.

ACUPRESSING:

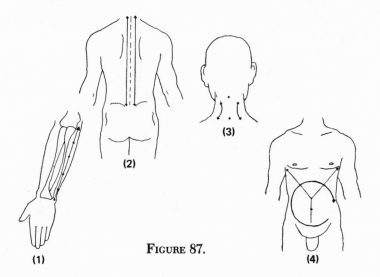

(1)   (2)   (3)   (4)

FIGURE 87.

20. NEPHRITIS AND CYSTITIS

PRESCRIPTION:

BODY POINTS: Shen-Shu (B 23), San-Yin-Chiao (SP 6), Pang-Kuan-Shu (B 28), Chi-Hai (JEN 6), Kuan-Yuan (JEN 4), Yin-Ling-Chuan (SP 9), Fu-Liu (K 7), Fei-Yang (B 58), Chung-Chi (JEN 3), Yang-Ling-Chuan (GB 34).

EAR POINTS: Kidney, bladder, adrenal gland, sympathetic, Shen-Men, subcortex.

METHOD OF TREATMENT: 1. Acute: Two treatments daily, *Dispersion.* 2. Improved case: Once daily, *Stimulation.* Treatment to continue as needed.

ACUPRESSING:

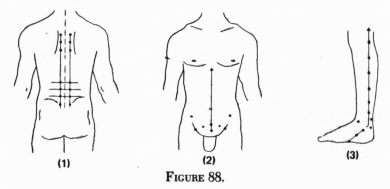

(1)   (2)   (3)

FIGURE 88.

21. IMPOTENCE AND PREMATURE EJACULATION

PRESCRIPTION:

BODY POINTS: Kuan-Yuan (JEN 4), San-Yin-Chiao (SP 6), Chung-Chi (JEN 3), Tsu-San-Li (S 36), Shen-Shu (B 23), Ming-Men (TU 4).

EAR POINTS: External genital organs, testis, adrenal gland, coccyx, bladder.

METHOD OF TREATMENT: Using *Stimulation,* one treatment daily, continuing as needed.

ACUPRESSING:

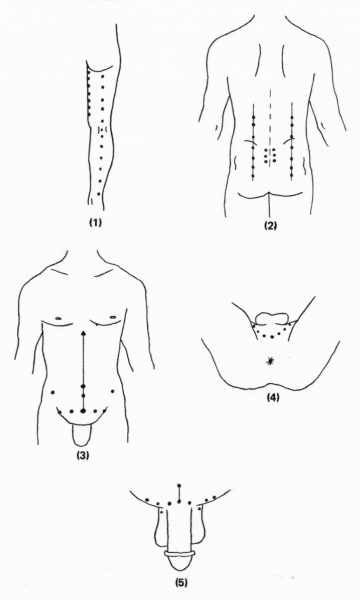

(1)

(2)

(3)

(4)

(5)

FIGURE 89.

22. DIABETES

PRESCRIPTION:

BODY POINTS: Pa-Chui-Hsa (new point—8th vertebra on the middle line of the back)-(TU 8_2), Yi-Shu (new point—1.5 tsun beside Pa-Chui-Hsa)-(B-17_2).

Associating with Shen-Shu (B 23), Ming-Men (TU 4), Fei-Shu (B 13), Jan-Ku (K 2), San-Yin-Chiao (SP 6), Kuan-Yuan (JEN 4).

EAR POINTS: Pancreas, liver, sympathetic, adrenal gland.

METHOD OF TREATMENT: Using *Stimulation,* one treatment daily, seven treatments making *one period of treatment. After three days of rest,* you may start a new period of treatment. Treatments may be continued for up to ten periods.

ACUPRESSING: For assistance only.

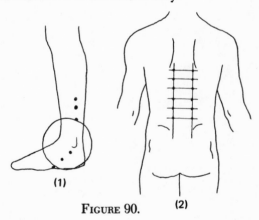

(1)

FIGURE 90.   (2)

23. PROSTATITIS:

PRESCRIPTION:

BODY POINTS: Chung-Chi (JEN 3), Yang-Ling-Chuan (GB 34), Kuan-Yuan (JEN 4), San-Yin-

Chiao (SP 36).

EAR POINTS: Prostate gland, internal secretion, kidney, subcortex.

METHOD OF TREATMENT: Using *Dispersion,* one or two treatments daily, continuing as needed.

ACUPRESSING: For assistance only.

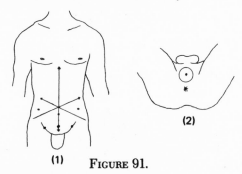

(1)   (2)   **FIGURE 91.**

24. HEMORRHAGIC DISEASES

PRESCRIPTION:

BODY POINTS: San-Yin-Chiao (SP 6), Hsueh-Hai (SP 10), Yung-Chuan (K 1), Ho-Ku (LI 4), Wai-Kuan (TH 5), Fei-Yang (B 58).

EAR POINTS: Liver, heart, spleen, sympathetic, internal secretion.

METHOD OF TREATMENT: One treatment every three days using *Stimulation.* Continue as needed.

ACUPRESSING: Not suitable.

25. ANEMIA AND APLASTIC ANEMIA

PRESCRIPTION:

BODY POINTS: Chung-Wan (JEN 12), Chu-Chih (LI 11), Nei-Kuan (HC 6), Lieh-Chueh (L 7), Ta-Chui (TU 14), Kan-Shu (B 18), Tan-Shu (B 19), Tsu-San-Li (S 36), San-Yin-Chiao (SP 6).

EAR POINTS: Liver, spleen, internal secretion, kidney, Shen-Men, small intestine.

METHOD OF TREATMENT: Using *Stimulation,* one treatment weekly, continuing as needed.

ACUPRESSING:

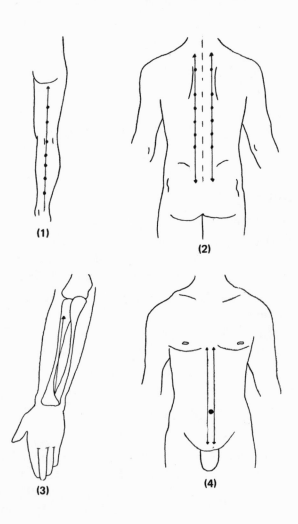

(1)

(2)

(3)

(4)

FIGURE 92.

26. FACIAL NERVE PARALYSIS

PRESCRIPTION:

BODY POINTS: Yang-pai (GB 14), Tai-Yang (temple), Ti-Tsang (S 4), Ying-Hsiang (LI 20), Ho-Ku (LI 4), Hsia-Kuan (S 7).
For pain, add Yi-Feng (TH 17)
For *amyotropic* or *agitans paralysis,* add Jen-Chung (YU 26), Chen-Chiang (YU 25), Chia-Che (S 6).

EAR POINTS: Back of head (occiput), mouth, eyes.

METHOD OF TREATMENT: 1. Acute: *Stimulation.* 2. Chronic: *Dispersion.* One treatment daily, continuing as needed.

ACUPRESSING: At least two treatments daily.

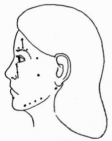

FIGURE 93.

27. TRIGEMINAL NEURALGIA

PRESCRIPTION:

BODY POINTS: 1. Pain on the first branch: Tsuan-Chu (B 2), Yang-Pai (GB 14), Ho-Ku (LI 4), Tsu-Lin-Chi (GB 41) and point of pain.
2. Pain on the second branch: Szu-Pai (S 2), Ying-Hsiang (LI 20), Ho-Ku (LI 4), Nei-Ting (S 44) and point of pain.
3. Pain on the third branch: Hsia-Kuan (S 7), Ti-Tsang (S 4), Wai-Kuan (TH 5), Tai-Chung (LV 3), and point of pain.

EAR POINTS: Cheek, lower palate, upper palate, back of head (occiput), Shen-Men.

METHOD OF TREATMENT: Dispersion, then *Stimulation.* Must leave needles in for more than 25 minutes. One treatment daily, continuing as needed.

ACUPRESSING:

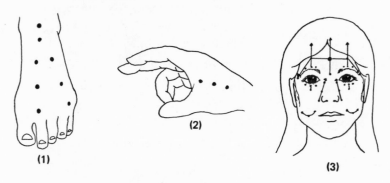

(1)   **(2)**   **(3)**

Figure 94.

28. INTERCOSTAL NEURALGIA

Prescription:

BODY POINTS: Chih-Kou (TH 6), Yang-Ling-Chuan (SP 9), Chi-Men (K 14), Shang-Chung (JEN 17).

For pain in the *liver area,* add Kan-Shu (B 18).

For pain in the *spleen area,* add Chang-Men (K 3), Tsu-San-Li (S 36).

(Note: Hua To's vertebral points should be associated.)

EAR POINTS: Chest, Shen-Men, back of head (occiput), subcortex.

METHOD OF TREATMENT: Using *Stimulation,* one treatment daily. Continue as needed.

ACUPRESSING:

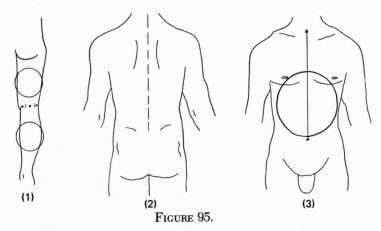

FIGURE 95.

29. SCIATICA

PRESCRIPTION:

BODY POINTS: Huan-Tiao (GB 30), Yang-Ling-Chuan (GB 34), Pai-Huan-Shu (B 30), Yin-Men (B 51), Cheng-Shan (B 57). Hsuan-Chung (GB 39) and Shen-Shu may be associated.

EAR POINTS: Buttock, coccyx, nervus ischiadicus, Shen-Men, adrenal gland.

METHOD OF TREATMENT: Using *Stimulation,* one treatment daily, continuing as needed.

ACUPRESSING:

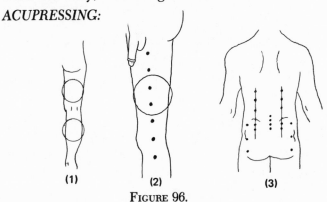

FIGURE 96.

30. INFANTILE PARALYSIS

PRESCRIPTION:

BODY POINTS: 1. *Upper limb:* Yang-lao (SI 6), Chu-chih (LI 11), Wai-kuan (TH 5), Tin-chuan (new point—½ tsun beside Ta-chui-TU 14).

2. *Lower limb:* Feng-shih (GB 31). Huan-tiao (GB 31), Yang-ling-chuan (GB 34), Wei-chung (B 54), Chu-chuan (K 8), Shang-chu-shih (S 37), Chieh-hsi (S 41), Tai-hsi (K 3), Shuan-chung (GB 39).

EAR POINTS: Subcortex, Shen-Men, back of head (occiput), adrenal gland, internal secretion.

METHOD OF TREATMENT: Once every day. *Dispersing,* then *Stimulating.*

ACUPRESSING:

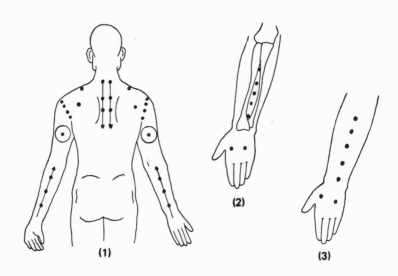

(2)

(1)

(3)

FIGURE 97. *Upper Limbs.*

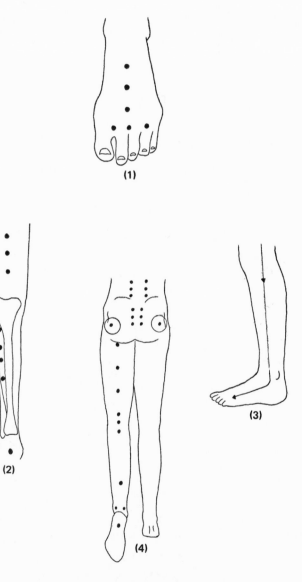

FIGURE 98. *Lower limbs.*

31. NEURITIS

PRESCRIPTION:

BODY POINTS: 1. Ascending: Kan-shu (B 18), Pi-shu (B 20), Chu-chih (LI 11), Wai-kuan (TH 5). 2. Descending: Kan-shu (B 18), Pi-shu (B 20), Tsu-san-li (S 36), San-yin-chiao (SP 6).

EAR POINTS: Disease area section, Shen-Men, adrenal gland, internal secretion.

METHOD OF TREATMENT: Once every day. *Stimulation.*

ACUPRESSING:

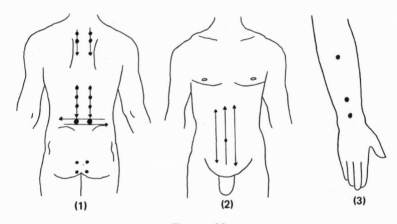

(1) (2) (3)

FIGURE 99.

32. STRUMA

PRESCRIPTION:

BODY POINTS: Ho-ku (LI 4), Tsu-san-li (S 36), Jen-yin (S 9), Tien-tu (JEN 22), Nei-kuan (P 6), San-yin-chiao (SP 6).

EAR POINTS: Shen-Men, subcortex, internal secretion, heart, pancreas, brain point.

METHOD OF TREATMENT: Once every day. *Dispersion, then Stimulation.*

ACUPRESSING:

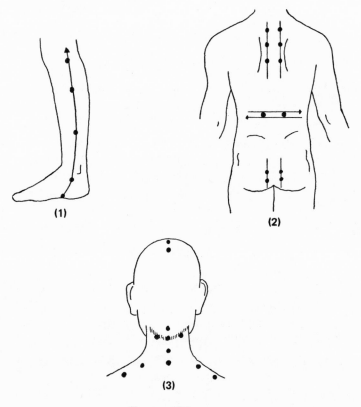

FIGURE 100.

17

GYNECOLOGY

1. DYSMENORRHEA

PRESCRIPTION:

BODY POINTS: 1. *Menstrual pain:* Kuan-yuan (Jen 4), Kuei-lai (S 29), Chu-chuan (LV 8).
2. *Premenstrual treatment:* Kuan-yuan (Jen 4), Kuei-lai (S 29), San-yin-chiao (SP 6), Chih-lao (B 32), Hueh-hai (SP 10), Hsin-chen (LV 2).

EAR POINTS: Uterus, internal secretion, sympathetic, Shen-Men.

METHOD OF TREATMENT: 1. Menstrual pain: Once daily. *Dispersion.*
2. Premenstrual treatment: Treatment should be in the week before menstruation, one treatment daily or every two days, using *Stimulation.* Three to four treatments may be repeated before menstruation.

ACUPRESSING:

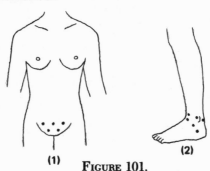

(1)   (2)

FIGURE 101.

2. PROLAPSE OF UTERUS

PRESCRIPTION:

BODY POINTS: Kuan-yuan (Jen 4), Chung-chi (Jen 3), Chu-ku (Jen 2), Wei-pao (strange point— 6 tsun beside Kuan-yuan (Jen 4), Chang-chiang (TU 1), Pai-hui (TU 20), Chih-lao (B 32), Ying-ling-chuan (SP 9).

EAR POINTS: Uterus, subcortex, external genital organ.

METHOD OF TREATMENT: Once daily. *Dispersed* then *Stimulated,* leaving needles for 30 minutes.

ACUPRESSING:

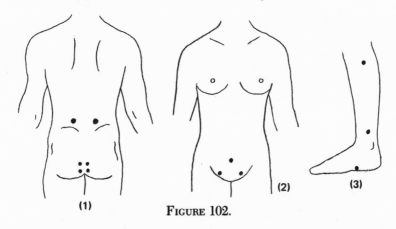

(1)   (2)   (3)

FIGURE 102.

3. FUNCTIONAL UTERINE HEMORRHAGE

PRESCRIPTION:

BODY POINTS: Tai-hsi (K 3), Kuan-yuan (Jen 4), Hseh-hai (SP 10), San-yin-chiao (SP 6), Fei-yang (B 58), Ti-chi (SP B).

EAR POINTS: Uterus, brain, point internal secretion, liver, spleen.

METHOD OF TREATMENT: Once daily or every other day. *Stimulation.*

ACUPRESSING:

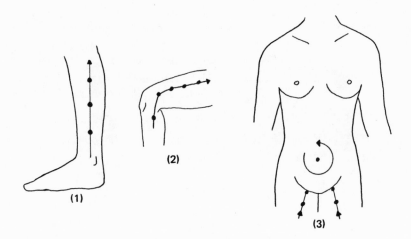

FIGURE 103.

4. LEUKORRHAGIA

PRESCRIPTION:

BODY POINTS: Kuei-lai (S 29), Chi-hai (Jen 5), San-yin-
chiao (SP 6), Hui-yin (Jen 1).

EAR POINTS: Uterus, internal secretion, Shen-Men, ovary.

METHOD OF TREATMENT: Once daily or every two
days. *Stimulation.*

ACUPRESSING:

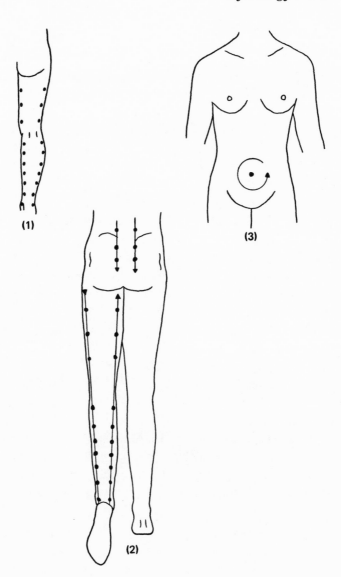

(1)

(2)

(3)

Figure 104.

18

SURGICAL DISEASE

1. ARTHRITIS

PRESCRIPTION:

BODY POINTS: 1. *Upper limb:* Chien-yu (LI 15), Chu-chih (LI 11), Wai-kuan (TH 5), Ho-ku LI 4).

2. *Lower limb:* Huan-tiao (GB 30), Chi-yen (strange point—2 tsun beside Tu-pi-S 35), Yang-ling-chuan (GB 34), Shuan-chung (GB 39), Che-hsi (S 41), Kun-lun (B 60).

3. *Vertebrae:* Using Tu-mo points, Hua-to-cha-chi-points, Ya-men (TU 15), Yin-men (B 51).

4. *Neck:* Hsa-kuan (S 7), Tin-hui (GB 2).

EAR POINTS: Shen-Men, kidney, internal secretion, back of head (occiput) and point of pain.

METHOD OF TREATMENT: Once or twice daily. *Stimulation.* After seven days, change to one treatment every other day, continuing as needed.

ACUPRESSING:

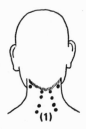

(1)

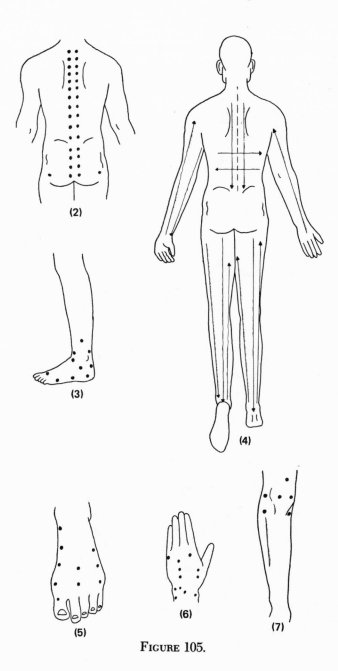

FIGURE 105.

2. MAMMITIS

PRESCRIPTION:

BODY POINTS: Ju-gung (S 18), Shan-chung (Jen 17), Ho-ku (LI 4), Shao-tse (SI 1), Tsu-lin-chi (GB 41), Nei-Ting (S 44).

EAR POINTS: Mammary gland, internal secretion, back of head (occiput).

METHOD OF TREATMENT: Once daily. *Dispersion.*

ACUPRESSING:

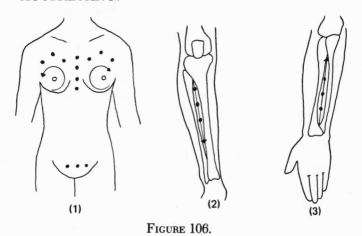

(1)   (2)   (3)

FIGURE 106.

3. ENTEREMPHRAXIS AND ENTEREPARALYSIS

PRESCRIPTION:

BODY POINTS: Tien-shu (S 25), Chi-Hai (Jen 6), Tsu-san-li (S 36), Kuan-yuan-shu (B 26), Chih-loa (B 32) Chu-chih (LI 11).

EAR POINTS: Sympathetic, large intestine, small intestine, subcortex.

METHOD OF TREATMENT: Once every three to four hours. *Dispersion.*

ACUPRESSING:

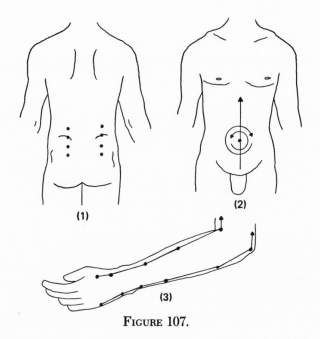

FIGURE 107.

4. CHOLECYSTITIS AND CHOLELITHIASIS

PRESCRIPTION:

BODY POINTS: Tan-shu (B 19), Chung-wan (Jen 12), Tsu-san-li (S 36).

For *pain,* add Yang-ling-chuan (GB 34), Ling-hsa (new point—2 tsun underneath Yang-ling-chuan, GB 34 on gallbladder meridian)

For *jaundice,* add Chih-yang (YU 9).

For *vomiting,* add Nei-kuan (P 6).

For *fever,* add Chu-chih (LI 11).

EAR POINTS: Gallbladder, sympathetic, Shen-Men, liver, duodenum.

METHOD OF TREATMENT: Once daily, ten treatments making a period of treatment. Rest two days, then take another period of treatment if needed. *Dispersion.*

PREVENTION: Needling body points as Tan-shu (B 19), Wan-ku (SI 4), Yang-ling-chuan (GB 34), Tsu-lin-chi (GB 41). Once or twice a week.

ACUPRESSING: For assistance only.

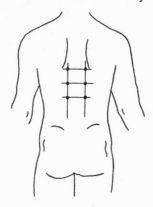

FIGURE 108.

5. *HEMORRHOIDS AND PROLAPSE OF ANUS*

PRESCRIPTION:

BODY POINTS: Chang-chiang (TU 1), San-yin-chiao (SP), Cheng-shan (B 57), Chih-lao (B 32).

EAR POINTS: Rectum, large intestine, subcortex, adrenal gland, spleen.

METHOD OF TREATMENT: Once daily. *Dispersion.*

ACUPRESSING:

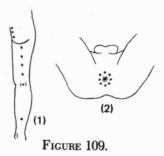

FIGURE 109.

6. RHINITIS

PRESCRIPTION:

BODY POINTS: Ying-Hsiang (LI 20), Ho-Ko LI 4), Yin-Tang (ST). Associate with Fei-Shu (B 13), Shen-Shu (B 23), San-Ying-Chiao (SP 6).

EAR POINTS: Lungs, inner nose, adrenal glands.

METHOD OF TREATMENT: Once daily, with seven treatments making one period of treatment.

ACUPRESSING:

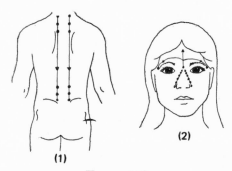

(2)

(1)

FIGURE 110.

7. DEAF-MUTISM

PRESCRIPTION:

BODY POINTS: Ya-Man (TU 15), Feng-Chih (GB 20), Yi-feng (TH 17), Ting-Kung (SI 19), Erh-Men (TH 21). Wai-Kuan (TH 6). Associate with Fei-Shu (B 13), Shen-Shu (B 23). Ying-Ling-Chuan (SP 9), Tsu-San-Li (S 36). Kuan-Yuan (Jen 4).

EAR POINTS: Not effective.

METHOD OF TREATMENT: Once daily, STIMULATION. May need a few periods of treatment.

ACUPRESSING: Not effective.

8. TONSILLITIS

PRESCRIPTION:

BODY POINTS: Ho-Ko (LI 4), Shao-Shaon (L 1), Tien-Chu (B 10), Nei-Ting (S 44).
For *fever,* add Chu-Chih (LI 11), Feng-Men (B 12).

EAR POINTS: Pharynx, Pien-Tao (tonsil).

METHOD OF TREATMENT: Once daily. *Dispersion* then *Stimulation.*

ACUPRESSING:

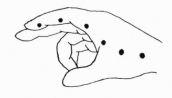

FIGURE 111.

19

THE FIVE-SENSES DISEASE

1. MYOPIA

PRESCRIPTION:

BODY POINTS: Ching-ming (B 1), Cheng-chi (S 1), Mei-chung (B 3), Yang-pai (GB 14), Szu-pai (S 2), Chen-ming (new point—½ tsun back side Pi-noe-LI 14), Yang-lao (SI 6), Tsu-san-li (S 36).

May be associated with Kan-shu (B 18), Shen-shu (B 23).

EAR POINTS: Kidney, liver, eye.

METHOD OF TREATMENT: Once daily, with ten treatments making one period of treatment. After three days of rest, you may start another period of treatment. *Stimulation.*

ACUPRESSING:

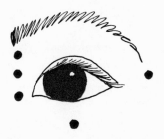

FIGURE 112.

2. HORDEOLUM

PRESCRIPTION:

BODY POINTS: Ching-ming (B 1), Tai-yang (temple), Ho-ku (LI 4), Feng-chih (GB 20).

EAR POINTS: Eyes, liver, spleen.

METHOD OF TREATMENT: Dispersion. Once every two days.

ACUPRESSING:

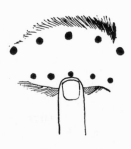

FIGURE 113.

3. GLAUCOMA

PRESCRIPTION:

BODY POINTS: Ching-ming (B 1), Tai-yang (temple), Chiu-hou (strange point—¼ tsun upper-outside direction beside Cheng-chi (S 1)), Ho-ku (LI 4).

For extreme pressure on the eyeball, add Hsin-chien (LV 2) or Tai-chung (LV 3).

For *headache,* add Wai-kuan (TH 16).

For *upset stomach,* add Tsu-san-li (S 36).

EAR POINTS: Eye, liver, kidney, and pressing points of pain.

METHOD OF TREATMENT: Once daily. *Stimulation.*

ACUPRESSING:

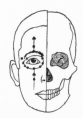

FIGURE 114.

4. CATARACT

PRESCRIPTION:

BODY POINTS: Ching-Ming (B 1), Yin-Tang, Tai-Yang (temple), Chiu-Hou, Cheng-Chi (S 1). Associate with Ho-Ko (LI 4), Wai-Kuan (TH 6).

EAR POINTS: Eye, liver, and pressing points of pain.

METHOD OF TREATMENT: Once daily. *Stimulation.*

ACUPRESSING: Same as No. 3.

5. OPTIC ATROPHY

PRESCRIPTION:

BODY POINTS: Ching-Ming (B 1), Chiu-Hou, Associate with Ho-Ko (LI 4), Wai-Kuan (TH 6).

EAR POINTS: Eye, liver.

METHOD OF TREATMENT: Once daily. *Stimulation.*

ACUPRESSING:

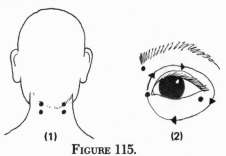

(1)   (2)

FIGURE 115.

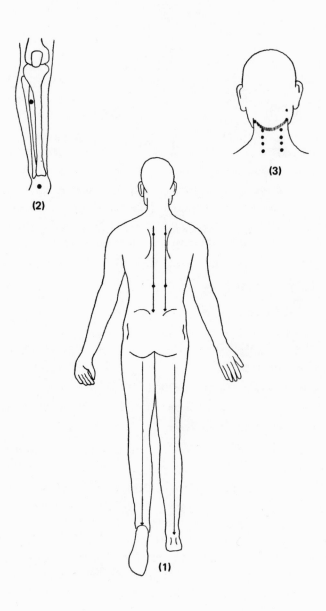

(2)

(3)

(1)

20

ACUPUNCTURE AND BEAUTY

The majority of people who are familiar with acupuncture and the various areas to which it has been applied often fail to realize the close relationship between acupuncture and beauty. Thinking of acupuncture only as a form of therapy, the idea that it can enhance and beautify the physical body is often a surprising revelation to many people. Acupuncture as a means of cultivating a beautiful body is perfectly logical if we first answer the question, "What exactly is beauty?"

Genuine beauty is a result of a deep inner vitality that permeates the entire body giving one a magnetic aura of dazzling radiance. Regardless of physical build, age, or body characteristics, this inner vitality will outshine deficiencies in any of these areas providing one has knowledge of, and persistence in, applying correct techniques that will cause the life energy to saturate all parts of the body. The final result is a natural glowing beauty that is sustained by the perfectly balanced flow of energy within the body.

Once the energy flow within the body has been balanced, artificial cosmetics and beauty aids, if they are needed at all, will be used to enhance or accentuate body features that one might wish to emphasize. Only in a body that is "starved" for life energy is there a need to overly mask oneself with cosmetics in an effort to cloak devitalized body features. Therefore, if a beautiful body is one's goal, a knowledge of practical acupuncture techniques that will rejuvenate the entire body is indispensable.

Healthy skin is possible for anyone whether the skin is at present oily or dry; and, rest assured, anyone can have silky, lustrous hair even if they're on the verge of baldness.

The condition of both the skin and the hair have a close relationship with the lungs. Actually, perspiration or skin breathing is an extension of the lungs' functioning. Therefore an evaluation of the energy balance within the lungs is the first step to beautifying the hair and skin. Diseased skin and lifeless hair are both a sure indication of an energy imbalance within the lungs; treating the points as illustrated will eventually eliminate all of these problems. The perfect functioning of the internal glands is also essential for healthy skin. Of special significance in the production of hormones is the thyroid gland; figure 116 (1) illustrates points on the neck which should be pressed to ensure a constant supply of vital hormones that will rejuvenate the entire body.

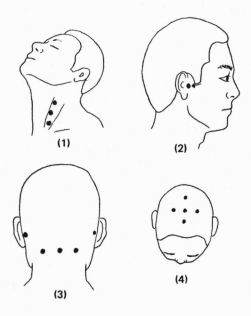

FIGURE 116.

The conservation of sexual energy will not only aid the condition of the skin but will also strengthen the entire body. When sexual energy has been conserved for an adequate length of time, a slow transformation of the body will commence. Therefore, regulating the menstrual cycle is essential for women, and men are advised not to dissipate their energy in unnecessary ejaculations.

Balancing the energy within the entire body will automatically provide hair cells with adequate nourishment to grow hair with a beautiful, natural sheen even in the most seemingly hopeless cases.

So called "crows-feet" and wrinkles around the eyes can be eliminated by pressing the points illustrated in figure 117 and by massaging around the eyes as indicated in figure 118. Notice the direction of the massage in that it differs from the massage that people generally use upon awakening. Rather than causing the muscles to droop, as with prolonged use of the outward directional massage, the inward directional massage will tonify the entire area surrounding the eyes.

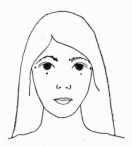

FIGURE 117.

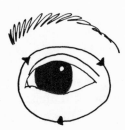

FIGURE 118.

A few minutes daily spent on the following exercise is a guarantee of keeping the original set of teeth in top condition for a lifetime. Stimulate the gums by massaging the cheeks atop the entire bottom and lower gums as shown in figure 119. Another way to stimulate the gums is to grit the teeth 36 times upon arising. Finally, when urinating or during the expulsion of fecal matter, grit the teeth tightly; for it is during these moments that the entire system is "loosened" or relaxed and therefore very vulnerable.

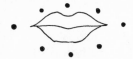

FIGURE 119.

With respect to weight problems, a diagnosis and adjustment of the digestive system is mandatory. If one is overweight, it means over-eating, or that the digestive system is absorbing every particle of food eaten, or both. Application of dispersal techniques will regulate the overactive digestive system and will simultaneously curb the appetite. For those who are underweight, the opposite of the preceding must be applied. Specific points to be treated are listed earlier in Part III.

To counteract the aging process, special attention should be given to the entire nervous system. Not only will an acute sensitivity to the external environment be maintained, but also all the organs of the body will be enlivened with vital force. Pain in the shoulders and back indicates a loss of suppleness in the joints that is indicative of age. Figure 120 illustrates the points to be treated to stimulate the flow of energy to the nervous system.

To cultivate a beautiful body should be a pleasant endeavor as long as one's life may last. Natural beauty need never be the outcome of tedious effort, but rather the natural outcome of simple life-promoting exercises. The techniques described in this chapter, if faithfully followed, will provide a constant level of energy that will sustain the bodily processes throughout life.

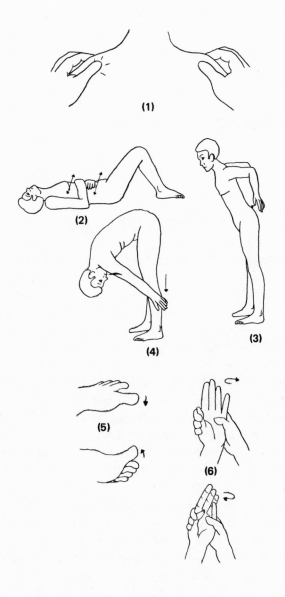

FIGURE 120.

21

ACUPUNCTURE AND ADDICTION

The nature of drug addiction is of such complexity that no true solution to this problem has yet been discovered. At present there are almost as many methods of solving the drug problem as there are variations on the problem itself. Whether the addiction is viewed as psychological or physiological, the end results of present-day treatments have been discouraging.

Treatment from a physiological basis, i.e. with methadone, merely replaces one drug with the use of another. True, methadone is less harmful than heroin, but *all drugs and chemicals will ultimately have a harmful effect on the body's internal organs and their functions* if used over a prolonged period of time.

Psychological counseling can be effective in breaking drug habits in which, of course, the dependence is basically psychological. Long term counseling is generally necessary and it is often difficult to maintain a constant, high level of motivation on the part of the addict to change his life style. Consequently, there are often many relapses and sometimes an abandonment of the entire project.

How then can the problem of drug addiction be effectively dealt with once it has become firmly established in one's life. Regardless of whether the addiction is physiological or psychological, it is first necessary to recognize the underlying factor or cause of the addiction that is common to both. In either case there is an uncontrollable urge in the mind of the addict that mercilessly gnaws at him until the drug is obtained and peace of mind is once again regained—as temporary as that might be. Once the effect of the drug wears off, again the desires prompt the addict into action until the mind-soothing drug is again obtained. A diagnosis made upon an addict at the time of his greatest desire for a drug will reveal a highly agitated state of energy within the body.

Chinese medicine offers a unique form of therapy for the elimination of self-destructive addictions regardless of the form they take—physiological or psychological. The neutralization of the desires that prompt one to obtain the drug is the first step of therapy. Whenever the irresistible urge for the drug arises within the addict, needles are inserted to balance the agitated energy flow within the body. Balancing the energy takes the place of the drug by naturally soothing the mind, and the desire that previously goaded the addict in a frantic chase after the drug is diminished and eventually rendered powerless. The necessary changes in life style can easily be carried out by a person who sincerely wants freedom from his habit while undergoing therapy.

Curing a person addicted to drugs can be a lengthy process depending on the type of addiction and the length of time the drug has been taken. In many cases I've had to administer treatments three times a day for a week to curb the desire. As recurrence of the desire lessens, so also do the number of treatments. Hospitalization is usually necessary in serious cases.

To see a human being become a slave to his desires rather than a master of them is a pitiful sight that should evoke compassion in the heart of anyone. My experiences in curing drug addicts has given me the firm conviction that no case of addiction is either permanent or hopeless.

BIBLIOGRAPHY

Academy of Traditional Chinese Medicine, *An Outline of Chinese Acupuncture.* San Francisco: China Books & Periodicals, 1975.

———, *Acupuncture Anaesthesia.* San Francisco: China Books & Periodicals, 1975.

Acupuncture & Moxibustion Editorial Committee, *Basic Acupuncture Techniques.* San Francisco: Basic Medicine Books, 1973.

Austin, Mary, *Acupuncture Therapy,* 2nd ed. New York: ASI Pubs, Inc., 1972.

———, *The Textbook of Acupuncture Therapy,* rev. 2nd ed. New York: ASI Pubs, Inc. 1975.

Chan, Pedro, *Wonders of Chinese Acupuncture.* Alhambra, Calif.: Borden Pub. Co.

Lavier, J., *Points of Chinese Acupuncture,* 2nd rev. ed. New York: Samuel Weiser, 1974.

Lawson-Wood, D., and Lawson-Wood, J., *Acupuncture Handbook,* 2nd ed. New York: British Book Center, 1973.

———, *Five Elements of Acupuncture and Chinese Massage.* New York: British Book Center, 1973.

———, *Multi-Lingual Atlas of Acupuncture.* New York: British Book Center, 19,5.

Lowe, William C., *Introduction to Acupuncture Anaesthesia.* Flushing, N.Y.: Medical Examination Pub. Co., 1973.

Mann, Felix, *Acupuncture,* rev. ed. New York: Random House, 1973.

———, *Acupuncture, the Ancient Chinese Art of Healing.* Gloucester, Mass.: Peter Smith.

———, *Acupuncture,* rev. ed. New York: Random House, 1972.

Matsumoto, Teruo, *Acupuncture for Physicians.* Springfield, Ill.: C. C. Thomas, 1974.

Tan, Leong T., *Acupuncture Therapy: Current Chinese Practice.* Philadelphia: Temple U. Press, 1976.

Wei-Ping, Wu, *Chinese Acupuncture.* New York: Samuel Weiser, 1973.

Wen, Hui, and Wei-Kang, Fu, *Acupuncture Anaesthesia.* Hazelwood, Missouri: Great Wall Press, 1972.

INDEX